You Can Be Beautiful

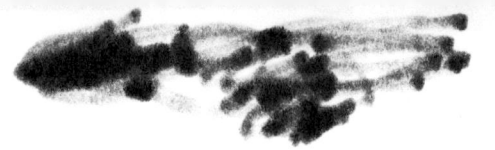

You Can Be Beautiful

With Beauty That Never Fades

Lottie Beth Hobbs

HARVEST PUBLICATIONS
P.O. Box 8456   Fort Worth, Texas 76124

Books by Lottie Beth Hobbs

Choosing Life's Best —
 The success plan of Proverbs
Daughters of Eve —
 Strength for today from women of yesterday
Victory Over Trials —
 Encouragement from the life of Job
 (originally titled *More Precious Than Gold*)
Your Best Friend —
 The privilege of friendship with Christ
If You Would See Good Days —
 Help for daily decisions
 (originally titled *Out of This World*)
You Can Be Beautiful —
 With beauty that never fades

25th English printing
ISBN 0-913838-01-2

Copyright 1959, 1990

HARVEST PUBLICATIONS
Fort Worth, Texas 76124

Cover art by Peggy Hobbs, copyright 1990

ALL RIGHTS RESERVED. No portion of this book may be reproduced in any form without written permission from the publisher.

Foreword

BEAUTY has always been of universal interest to women and men alike. It is possible to develop beauty that is captivating, a calm loveliness of soul that is both sacred and compelling. God tells us how. He has given the mirror for the soul, which enables us to see our imperfections and needs, and he has given all the beauty ingredients and instructions for application. The purpose of this series of lessons is to consider the divine beauty plan.

This life is the dressing-room to prepare for eternity. Some day all earthly accomplishments will fade into nothingness; all material wealth will lose its value; physical bodies, whether beautiful or otherwise, will decay. But there is a part of us which will never die. Life's most urgent task is to keep the inner being well-groomed, free from the stains of sin, ready to appear before the Great Judge of the only beauty contest that really counts. How shall we look as we appear before him? How do we look to him now?

> Though thy name be spread abroad
> Like winged seed from shore to shore,
> What thou art before thy God
> That thou art and nothing more.

Questions are given at the close of each chapter for those who wish to review their study. Their use is optional, of course. The answers are found within the chapter text. The thought questions are given to stimulate further study or discussion on related topics. All Scripture quotations are from the King James Version, unless otherwise stated.

Though limited space makes it necessary to omit many things, all basic requirements in God's plan for spiritual beauty are included, both positive and negative. It takes both. So we shall study the positive traits which enhance inward beauty and those negative traits which destroy it.

Although these lessons are especially designed for women, the principles certainly apply to everyone. May the Lord bless their use as all of us strive to groom our souls for that inevitable day when each shall stand before the great white throne for the final examination. May we appear beautiful and blameless, prepared to receive the eternal diploma: "Well done, thou good and faithful servant: enter thou into the joy of thy Lord."

—LOTTIE BETH HOBBS

Fort Worth, Texas

Contents

I. Portrait of a Lovely Life — 7

II. "The Beauty of Holiness" — 14

III. The Power That Cleanses — 20

IV. Royal Robes for the Heart — 26

V. Disposition Diseases — 33

VI. A Matter of Life and Death — 40

VII. For Daily Application — 48

VIII. "Unspotted from the World" — 55

IX. "Keep Me from Presumptuous Sins" — 62

X. Your Siamese Twins — 69

XI. The Adorning of Sympathy — 76

XII. "Awake Thou That Sleepest" — 82

XIII. Sharing God's Beauty Plan — 89

I

Portrait of a Lovely Life

CHRIST is the central figure of all time. As the hub is to the wheel, so is he to the Bible and to all history. When the blackness of sin engulfed all humanity, a cross was lighted on Calvary's hill; and its rays stream down through the centuries assuring us that God loves, God cares, and God redeems. The very foundations of the world were shaken and the course of civilization was changed by this solitary life of the Son of God.

Just as you may look at several poses of your baby's picture and see different aspects which make up the whole of personality, so we may look at four different views of the loveliest life the world has ever known. Matthew pictured for the Jews a King and his kingdom. Mark pictured the wonder-working Man of Action. Luke portrayed the Ideal Man for the Greeks, who so admired manhood. John pictured God's Son, the embodiment of the Father, the Universal Saviour.

I. "TO BEHOLD THE BEAUTY OF THE LORD."

The Psalmist said: *"One thing have I desired . . . to behold the beauty of the Lord"* (Psalms 27:4). Men have always longed to see God. A little girl prayed: "God, let me see your face when I talk to you." Those of Old Testament times had God's word, but they had never seen him. One reason Christ came into the world was to show us the Father. Beholding that loveliness enshrined in the life of Jesus of Nazareth gives us a picture of the Father (Jno. 14:9).

The life of Christ bears testimony that *true loveliness can be achieved regardless of physical characteristics.* Though we have no description of his physical traits, and some have thought Isaiah 53:2 might indicate that he was not handsome, yet his real beauty has never been equaled.

II. A LIFE WITH A PURPOSE.

Jesus came into the world to save sinners. All other activities were incidental as his life was centered around this one glorious goal. This gave him spiritual poise, the ability to meet every blow of life unwaveringly and triumphantly. Temptation, loneliness, sorrows, physical fatigue, false brethren, wicked leaders, religious indifference — none of these things could deter him from his life's purpose or cause him to lose his spiritual balance.

The abundant life which Christ came to bring his followers (Jno. 10:10) cannot be achieved by aimless drifting and a life consumed with trifles. Neither can it be achieved if our lives are centered on the wrong goal. "Let us hear the conclusion of the whole matter: Fear God, and keep his commandments: for this is the whole duty of man" (Eccl. 12:13). This sums up not only the right goal in life but also the formula for abundant living. Since we have only one life, wisdom demands that we appraise our present goals and consider what will be the end of all our labors.

III. OBEDIENCE AND RESPECT FOR AUTHORITY.

Jesus was obedient to his parents (Luke 2:51). A man once advertised: "Wanted to work in my shop — a boy who obeys his parents." This lesson, learned early, will help promote a lifetime of peace and happiness. A failure to learn it will foster maladjustment and frustration; for the principle of obedience to authority is carried into every realm of life — obedience to school authorities, civil laws, elders, husband, employer, and God.

"Lo, I come to do thy will, O God" (Heb. 10:9). Christ's obedience and subjection to the authority of the Father permeated his whole life. He kept God's law and taught others the necessity of doing so (Heb. 5:8, 9).

IV. TENDERNESS AND COMPASSION.

Only weak characters are cruel. Our Lord was strong enough to be tender. This was shown by his feeling for children (Luke 18:15-17), and by his love for the sinful and the outcast (Luke 7:36-50; John 4:7-30). He sympathized with the sorrowing. His heart yearned to help even those who rejected him, and the depth of his feeling is revealed as he exclaimed over the lost multitudes of a great city: "O Jerusalem, Jerusalem . . . how often would I have gathered thy children together, as a hen doth gather her brood under her wings, and ye would not!" (Luke 13:34).

So yielding was Christ's great heart toward the welfare of others that the divine record specifies three times that he wept. Tears can be sacred and often manifest strength rather than weakness.

V. FIRMNESS AND CONVICTION.

Loving and tender, *yet the Son of God is also called the Lion of Judah;* and such he was when divine truth was challenged. The spineless tolerance sometimes attributed to him was no part of the spirit of Christ. He taught that truth is fixed and unchangeable and that obedience to it is an absolute necessity.

So many of his teachings bear testimony to this. Listen to the uncompromising firmness of some of the statements which fell from his lips: "For if ye believe not that I am he, ye shall die in your sins" (Jno. 8:24). "I am the way, the truth, and the life: no man cometh unto the Father, but by me" (Jno. 14:6). "Except ye repent, ye shall all likewise perish" (Luke 13:3). "Because strait is the gate, and narrow is the way, which leadeth unto life, and few there be that find it" (Matt. 7:14).

If we are to follow the lovely pattern, *we must have strength enough to stand for the truths of God.* No doubt many today would have told Christ: "Your preaching is too hard and entirely too narrow." Nevertheless, no amount of pressure or temptation ever led him to compromise truth.

VI. A MAN OF SORROWS WHO SPREAD JOY TO OTHERS.

Though physical strength may be measured by how much we can carry, *spiritual strength is sometimes measured by how much we can bear.* Through a turbulent life and an unjust death, Christ set a heroic example which has in all centuries fortified trouble-tossed hearts to brave the storms of suffering, persecution, and despair.

> His beauty, tho' bleeding and circled with thorns,
> Is then most exceeding, for grief Him adorns.
> —J. E. Rankin

The sublimest joys can be experienced only by those who have borne the weightiest griefs, for the soul bruised the deepest by sorrow can hold the truest happiness. Some of the loftiest masterpieces of art, music, and literature were conceived in broken hearts. Christ, the man of sorrows who brought joy to the world — the only real joy the world can know — admonished his followers: "Rejoice, rejoice." Christians today who carry crosses almost unbearably heavy can "rejoice, because your names are written in heaven" (Luke 10:20) and can be a source of joy to others.

VII. CLOSE COMMUNION WITH THE FATHER.

Christ's deep sense of need for communion with the Father led him to frequent prayer; for instance, after his baptism, before selecting the apostles, at the transfiguration, before his crucifixion, and on the cross with his last breath. When our knees become shaky, we can kneel on them. The strongest persons are those who realize a complete dependence upon God. Abraham Lincoln said: "I have been driven to my knees many times by a realization that I had no place else to go for help."

A constant consciousness of God will cause us to be mindful of his ever-present concern and care. Life is too complex for a person to handle it alone, but the Father who takes note of a fallen sparrow, feeds the ravens, and clothes the lilies is able and anxious to care for his children (Matt. 10:29-31; Matt. 6:28-30).

VIII. THE LIVING ALPHABET.

Jesus said, "I am Alpha and Omega" (Rev. 1:8) — the first and last letters of the Greek alphabet. In other words: "I am 'A' and 'Z' and all that is in between. I am everything." This masterpiece of imagery is almost beyond our finite comprehension. There is nothing in all God's planning that is not centered in Christ. Man has no spiritual need or

You Can Be Beautiful

longing which cannot be fulfilled by Christ. Man needs no example which is not furnished by Christ.

He "suffered for us, leaving us an example, that ye should follow his steps" (I Peter 2:21, 22). A Jewish boy once asked his Rabbi: "When our Messiah comes, what excellence will he have that Jesus of Nazareth did not possess?" Surely there could be none. In this lesson we have mentioned only a few of his traits of loveliness; he exemplifies every aspect of godliness discussed in the lessons to follow. Jesus was the Messiah, the one and only Messiah! Flowing from a pure heart were words of truth and salvation, deeds of comfort and helpfulness. He "went about doing good" (Acts 10:38) — this is his biography. Nothing is more admirable than a man with beauty of character, for being a Christian requires more real manhood than anything else in all the world. It cannot be done by weaklings.

"For in him dwelleth all the fulness of the Godhead bodily" (Col. 2:9). Christ is the Lamb of God, the Rose of Sharon, the Lily of the Valley, the Bright and Morning Star, the Bread of Life, the Good Shepherd. He is the Way, the Truth, and the Life. He is the Living Water; and after we take our little vessels to the ever-flowing stream and fill them to capacity, the source is still inexhaustible. He is the Light of the World, the Resurrection and the Life. Only through Christ is salvation for the sinful and rest for the weary. This Wonderful One invites us to be his friend, to commune with him, to partake of his strength, and to emulate his loveliness: "Behold I stand at the door, and knock: if any man hear my voice, and open the door, I will come in to him, and will sup with him, and he with me" (Rev. 3:20).

EXERCISE

1. What one thing was desired by the Psalmist? ....

....

2. Jesus said: "He that hath seen me hath seen ....

....,"

3. How does Eccl. 12:13 sum up the proper aims in life?
   ....
   ....

4. Christ became the "author of eternal salvation to all them that .... him."

5. We never outgrow the necessity of being subject to the authority of others. (T or F)

6. List three "I ams" given by Jesus: (1) ....
   (2) .... (3) ....

7. "Except ye ...., ye shall all likewise ....
   ...."

8. Quote Matt. 7:14: ....
   ....
   ....

9. Did Jesus teach that it doesn't matter what one believes, so long as he is honest and sincere? ....

10. Which indicates real strength: (1) a feeling of dependence upon God, or (2) a feeling of self-sufficiency?

11. List two examples Christ gave to show that God will care for his children: (1) .... (2) ....
    ....

12. How and why was Jesus compared to the alphabet? ....
    ....

13. Christ "suffered for us, leaving us an .... that ye should .... his ...."

FOR THOUGHT OR DISCUSSION

1. Since Christ had demonstrated superior knowledge and wisdom at the age of 12, why did he return to Nazareth and live subject to human parents?

2. Comment: a parent's failure to require obedience of a child is actually an injustice to the child.

3. To be like Christ, we must be friends of sinners. Does this mean that we are to choose our close friends among those who live wrong? Read also the warning given in I Cor. 15:33.

4. Examine yourself. What is your goal in life?

II

"The Beauty of Holiness"

FIVE different Scriptures, such as Psalms 96:9, refer to the "beauty of holiness." The loveliest person is that one whose life most nearly conforms to God's teachings and whose feet walk closest in the steps of the Perfect Pattern. The Bible refers to this as godliness, righteousness, or holiness.

I. REFLECTING THE RADIANCE OF HEAVEN.

An old sculptor in Europe made a model of a beautiful cathedral and placed it in his shop window. Many passed the window each day without noticing it, until one day he placed a light inside the model. Then everyone stopped in reverence to admire its beauty.

Christ said, "I am the light of the world." Then he said to his disciples: "Ye are the light of the world." As the light of God shines through human lives, all the world beholds the loveliness.

Godliness brings a little of heaven to this world and gives its glory to earthly lives. After Moses had been with God, his face literally shone, though Moses "wist not that his face shone."

> In holiness there is such a sparkling lustre, that whosoever beholds it must needs be astonished at it; nay, even those that oppose it cannot but admire it. Holiness is an excellent thing, a beautiful thing: it carries a graceful majesty along with it. —Spencer.

A holy life is one indisputable refutation to the atheist. A man once said: "I was an atheist, but I have concluded that the existence of God can be the only logical explanation of goodness and righteousness in the world." Man left to himself always goes downward, not upward; therefore, a righteous life is proof of an Elevating Force greater than man himself.

II. IT CAN BE DONE.

A lovely life must be deliberate; it never happens accidentally. Making the most of ourselves requires a lifetime of constant vigilance and diligence. Pleasing physical traits may be inherited, but true beauty must be acquired. A wise teacher often told her class of high school girls: "You may not be pretty at twenty, but at forty there is no excuse." Every admirable trait can be developed. We have within us the power to be all God intended. When we walk in righteousness, we appropriate an eternal power and fulfil an eternal purpose. God gives us life and a "do it yourself" kit. The rest is up to us.

All improvement — physical, mental, or spiritual — begins with a self-examination. The Psalmist said: "I thought on my ways, and turned my feet unto thy testimonies" (Psa. 119:59). The Prodigal Son made improvement only after he "came to himself" and faced the changes he needed to make (Luke 15:17).

God's word furnishes the mirror for the soul and is the only guide for spiritual improvement (Jas. 1:22-25). We are admonished to study it and give diligence to "show thyself approved unto God" (II Tim. 2:15). Most of Paul's writings were to sinners in the church, giving instructions for spiritual growth. As we look into the divine mirror, we must be honest with ourselves. Refusing to look will correct nothing. Neither will a refusal to admit the imperfections which we see.

The godly one described in the first Psalm is compared to a tree "planted" — a deliberate thing; "that bringeth forth fruit" — a blessing to others; whose "leaf shall not wither" — a lovely evergreen in spite of summer's heat or winter's storm; which "shall prosper" — the future is bright.

III. LOVELINESS THAT NEVER FADES.

What an encouraging thought! "But though our outward man perish, yet the inward man is renewed day by day" (II Cor. 4:16). Characteristics, whether good or bad, are intensified with age. Thus, grooming the heart is the only way to grow old gracefully. Spiritual beauty shines more gloriously than ever in age, sickness, and death. "For those who live right, and walk circumspectly, youth is opportunity, manhood is achievement, and old age a holy memory." —Gordon.

One of the loveliest things in the world is the aged Christian, grown sweet and mellow by a lifetime of association with the Master, facing the sunset of life with confidence and anticipation, leaving a legacy of good works and righteous influences. Indeed, the beauty of holiness is incomparable and eternal.

> An old age serene and bright,
> And lovely as a Lapland night
> Shall lead thee to thy grave.
>
> —Wordsworth

Proverbs 31:30 distinguishes for us *the traits that endure.* "Favor [popularity] is deceitful, and beauty [physical beauty] is vain: but a woman that feareth the Lord, she shall be praised." Many mothers work diligently to help daughters acquire the first two, favor and beauty, with little thought for teaching fear of the Lord. A life not founded upon the commandments of God will eventually crumble, leaving only heartache and despair. A compliance with divine law develops a beauty that is deep, enduring, satisfying, and worthy of the honor and praise of God and mankind. Such a one becomes also a source of strength to so many others — "strength and honor are her clothing" (Prov. 31:25).

IV. THE TWO OF YOU.

"But though our outward man perish, yet the inward man is renewed day by day" (II Cor. 4:16). Surely we understand that each of us is two beings, the outward and the inward. "For the Lord seeth not as man seeth; for man looketh on the outward appearance, but the Lord looketh on the heart" (I Sam. 16:7). Do these Scriptures mean that God has no concern with our "outward man"? Not at all.

God is the Creator of all beauty, even though Satan may employ some things to his advantage. The indescribable wonders of nature, alive with exciting colors, emanate from his creative hand, and he formed the physical loveliness of humanity.

The Lord had enough interest to describe the physical appearance of many characters and often mentions their beauty. He has always understood mankind's interest in the outward being. As a matter of fact, such is even one mark of sanity. One of the symptoms of severe mental illness is a complete unconcern over physical appearance. The worthy woman loved beauty and created for her family and herself garments of loveliness (Prov. 31:21, 22).

God has always been *concerned with the clothing of the body* — so much so that he himself made clothing for Adam and Eve (Gen. 3:21), and he is concerned about apparel today (I Tim. 2:9).

God has always been *concerned with the care of the body*, for it is the temple of the Holy Spirit (I Cor. 3:16, 17; 6:19, 20). Christ realized the need of caring for the body and at times withdrew from the multitudes to rest, despite his urgent work. The wise woman "girdeth her loins with strength, and strengtheneth her arms" (Prov. 31:17). She needs physical strength for the tasks ahead. So many are depending upon her.

V. KEEPING THE PROPER BALANCE.

"*Whose adorning, let it not be that outward adorning* of plaiting of the hair, and of wearing of gold, or of putting on of apparel; but let it be the hidden man of the heart, in that which is not corruptible, even the ornament of a meek and quiet spirit, which is in the sight of God of great price" (I Peter 3:3, 4). Does this forbid one to plait the hair or wear gold? If so, it would also forbid the wearing of any clothes — "not the putting on of apparel." Therefore, we must conclude that the real meaning is that we must keep the outward adorning in its proper relationship, understanding at all times that the grooming of the soul is our vital task. The same principle applies also to I Timothy 2:9, 10. The adorning of "good works" must surely take precedence over physical grooming.

Physical beauty can be used as a God-given blessing. For instance, Esther's beauty was used to advance God's cause. The same has been true of others. But how shabby and repulsive is the fair countenance which cloaks an evil heart. If godliness accompanies physical beauty, one is doubly blessed; but if vice is associated with it, it becomes the soul's liability. What good is an apple with rosy skin, if worms have devoured its heart? God describes David as a comely person, but our real admiration for him stems from the fact that he was a man after God's own heart — this pictures his noble soul.

EXERCISE

1. We can be "the light of the world" only as we reflect the light of ....
2. Turning your feet unto the Lord's testimonies begins with ....
3. What is the mirror for the soul? .... Can anything else show us how we actually look to God? ....
4. We are commanded to "........................... to show thyself .... unto God."
5. Can man perish and be renewed at the same time? .... Scripture: ....
6. How can one grow old gracefully? ....
7. Which three traits are mentioned in Prov. 31:30? (1) .... (2) .... (3) .... What is said of each one?
8. List two Scriptures which show that God is interested in what we wear: (1) .... (2) ....
9. Christian women are to "adorn themselves in .... apparel."
10. The body is the temple of the .... What will happen to those who destroy that temple? ....

YOU CAN BE BEAUTIFUL

11. The wise woman "girdeth her loins with ....,
and strengtheneth her ...."
12. With what did the worthy woman clothe her family? ....
....
13. Yet the most important adorning must be the "........................
.... man of the ...."

FOR THOUGHT OR DISCUSSION

1. Think of the most godly person you know. Does he or she have one spiritual trait that you could not acquire, if you were willing to put forth the effort?
2. What did the Prodigal Son have to do before he could ever better his own condition?
3. Discuss the comparison which James uses to show the folly of recognizing our spiritual imperfections and then doing nothing.

III

The Power That Cleanses

EVERY woman recognizes the relationship between cleansing and beauty, which makes it easy to understand that the first and basic requirement of spiritual beauty is a continual application of the divine cleansing agent for the soul.

I. GOD'S MORAL GOVERNMENT DEMANDS ATONEMENT FOR SIN.

The parent or government which does not hold subordinates responsible for wrong-doing will soon find a state of chaos. When God created man in his own image and showered upon him every imaginable blessing, *he also gave him a law to be obeyed* and the ability to choose to obey or disobey. Man sinned, and justice demanded that he be destroyed for his wrong-doing; but God's supreme devotion prompted him to make provisions for man to live eternally. This is the story of the Bible — a love story, the story of a loving Creator and the redemption of his most beloved creatures.

"*For all have sinned,* and come short of the glory of God" (Rom. 3:23). Each person who has reached the age of responsibility has committed sins which stain his soul and bar him from heaven, for "there shall in no wise enter into it any thing that defileth" (Rev. 21:27). This being true, the most serious task facing each person is to cleanse his soul from sin and to keep himself continually unspotted and ready to enter eternity. What has the power to remove sin?

II. THE BLOOD OF CHRIST IS THE ONLY CLEANSER FOR THE SOUL.

Christ's blood atonement for man's sin is the central theme of the Bible, a crimson thread running from Genesis to Revelation. It has been said: "The Bible is vascular; no matter where you prick it, it bleeds." Salvation is inseparably connected with the blood of Christ.

Though sin made the cross and plaited the crown of thorns, it was divine love that yielded to the pain and shame *to bring redemption to all who would be washed in the crimson flow.* "For this is my blood of the new testament, which is shed for many for the remission of sins" (Matt. 26:28). "In whom we have redemption through his blood, the forgiveness of sins" (Eph. 1:7). Concerning Christ it is said: "For thou wast slain, and hast redeemed us to God by thy blood" (Rev. 5:9). Entrance into heaven will be granted those who have "washed their robes, and made them white in the blood of the Lamb" (Rev. 7:14).

> When the Bridegroom cometh will your robes be white,
> Pure and white in the blood of the Lamb?
> Will your soul be ready for the mansions bright,
> And be washed in the blood of the Lamb?
>
> —E. A. Hoffman

III. NO OTHER MEANS OF CLEANSING.

The foregoing Scriptures show the absolute necessity of the blood of Christ in the salvation of mankind. This being true, the guilt of sin can never be removed:

By the philosophies of men.

By simply denying that sin exists. Some feel that sin can be eliminated by merely refusing to recognize it as evil.

By following the moral and ethical teachings of Christ alone, while rejecting the power of his blood. Many attempt to do this today, but to deny Christ's blood atonement for sin would destroy the very core of the Bible and nullify its entire meaning.

By a transformed life and good works alone. Clean living and good works are necessary, but such do not remove the guilt of sin. If so, then Christ died in vain; for moral goodness was practiced before Christ came into the world. No, a social gospel is not enough.

IV. THE OLD TESTAMENT SHADOW OF CHRIST'S DEATH.

The reason for the use of blood in atonement for sin is given in Leviticus 17:11. "For the life of the flesh is in the blood; and I have given it to you upon the altar to make an atonement for your souls: for it is the blood that maketh an atonement for the soul." God's goodness and love prompted him to accept the life of the animal as a substitute for the life of the sinner. "It is not possible that the blood of bulls and of goats should take away sins" (Heb. 10:4), but such was a shadow, or type, of the blood atonement of Christ and served to impress the fact that "without shedding of blood is no remission" (Heb. 9:22). God spent centuries schooling mankind to understand this principle.

During the patriarchal age, animal sacrifices were made by Abel, Noah, Abraham, and many others.

Under the law of Moses, God gave detailed instructions concerning animal sacrifices. One of the many observances was the annual day of atonement, which is described in Leviticus 16. The high priest washed himself and dressed in white linens; then he offered a bullock for himself and his family. Two goats were brought, and lots were cast to determine which one would be sacrificed as a sin offering. Upon the other goat, called the scapegoat, the high priest laid his hands and confessed the sins of all Israel. Then the goat was sent into the wilderness carrying the sins away. Such typified the redemptive work of Jesus.

Christ's atonement for our sins was *foretold in many prophecies,* such as: "The Lord hath laid on him the iniquity of us all" (Isaiah 53:4-7). John the Baptist, the man sent by God to herald Christ's work to the world, said: "Behold the Lamb of God which taketh away the sin of the world!" (Jno. 1:29).

V. HOW CAN WE CONTACT CHRIST'S CLEANSING BLOOD?

Though Christ shed his blood for all (Heb. 2:9), the majority of the world will be lost (Matt. 7:13, 14). Why? Because comparatively few will appropriate the saving blood to their own souls. The most powerful cleansing agent in the world is of no value unless applied. Surely God tells how to apply Christ's saving blood.

We must believe the gospel of Christ, for it is "the power of God unto salvation." What does it mean to believe the gospel? One must believe the facts of the gospel: ". . . how that Christ died for our sins according to the Scriptures; and that he was buried, and that he arose again the third day according to the Scriptures" (I Cor. 15:1-4). One must understand and believe that Christ is truly the Son of God (Jno. 8:24).

Understanding that we are sinners and that Christ loved us enough to die for us should surely prompt *repentance of sins.* Repentance is a change of mind which is produced by godly sorrow for sin and is followed by a reformation of life. Such is necessary for salvation (Acts 17:30).

We must be willing to *confess before men the faith in our hearts,* to confess that we "believe that Jesus Christ is the Son of God" (Acts 8:37).

But faith, repentance, and confession alone will not cleanse the soul from sin. A forceful example of this fact is seen in the life of Saul of Tarsus, later known as the apostle Paul. After he had believed in Christ and had become so penitent that he fasted for three days, he was still in his sins. His faith and penitence had not removed the guilt of sin, for God sent Ananias to tell him to "arise, and be baptized, and wash away thy sins" (Acts 22:16). This testifies conclusively that Saul was still in his sins until he contacted the cleansing blood of Christ in the act of baptism. This harmonizes perfectly with Romans 6:3, 4: "Know ye not, that so many of us as were baptized into Jesus Christ were baptized into his death? Therefore we are buried with him by baptism into death. . ."

Thus, baptism is the final step which takes away the guilt of sin. Until such is done with an understanding heart, we still have the guilt of sin upon our souls (Rom. 6:17, 18). Christ shed his blood in his death; and when penitent believers obey the form of his death, burial, and resurrection, they contact the saving blood and enter into Christ (Gal. 3:27). When we are cleansed by Christ's blood, God adds us to his church; for the church is that body of people purchased by the blood of Christ (Acts 20:28).

VI. A CONTINUAL CLEANSING NECESSARY.

After baptism into Christ's death removes the guilt of all past sins, *we must still continually cleanse our souls.* How is this done? "But if we walk in the light, as he is in the light, we have fellowship one with another, and the blood of Jesus Christ his Son cleanseth us from all sin" (I Jno. 1:7-10). What does it mean to walk in the light? To walk according to the commandments of God. All Christians fail at times to do this and must again have the stain of sin removed.

God gives a law of pardon to erring Christians, a means of cleansing. A Christian who had sinned was told to "repent and pray" (Acts 8:22). Also, "If we confess our sins, he is faithful and just to forgive us our sins, and to cleanse us from all unrighteousness" (I Jno. 1:9). "Confess your faults one to another, and pray one for another, that ye may be healed" (Jas. 5:16). Thus, sin in the life of a child of God must be removed by repentance, confession, and prayer.

EXERCISE

1. God used blood to atone for man's sins because: "The .... of the flesh is in the blood."
2. The animal sacrifices of the Old Testament were a .... of the blood sacrifice of ...."
3. "Without shedding of blood is no ...."
4. "For all have ...., and come .... of the glory of God."
5. Those granted an entrance into heaven will be those who have "................ their robes and made them white in the .... of the ...."

YOU CAN BE BEAUTIFUL

6. Did Jesus state why his blood was to be shed? ....
   Scripture: ....
7. List four futile efforts of man to atone for sins:
   (1) ....
   (2) ....
   (3) ....
   (4) ....
8. What did the Lord lay on Jesus? ....
9. If Christ shed his blood for everybody, why will not everybody be saved? ....
10. The facts of the gospel are the ...., ... and .... of Christ.
11. Saul of Tarsus was told to "arise and be .... and .... away thy ...."
12. We contact Christ's blood when we are "................. with him by .... into death."
13. "In whom we have redemption through his ...., the forgiveness of sins." "In whom" refers to .... How does one get into Christ? ....
14. What did Christ purchase with his blood? ....
15. How can we live in a constant state of cleansing? ....
....

FOR THOUGHT OR DISCUSSION

1. Inasmuch as God has demanded repentance as a condition of salvation in every dispensation, then is it not logical to conclude that any sin unrepented of remains unforgiven? Does this apply to Christians also?
2. Are not modernists inconsistent in claiming to be Christians on the one hand and denying Christ's blood atonement on the other hand?

IV

Royal Robes for the Heart

"PUT on therefore, as the elect of God, holy and beloved..." (Col. 3:12-14); and in this citation Paul gives a list of the royal robes for the heart. Other lovely garments are specified by Peter: "And besides this, giving all diligence, add to your faith virtue; and to virtue, knowledge; and to knowledge, temperance; and to temperance, patience; and to patience, godliness; and to godliness, brotherly kindness, and to brotherly kindness, charity" (love, A.S.V.) (II Peter 1:5-9). Those who walk by the Spirit will be robed in "love, joy, peace, long-suffering, gentleness, goodness, faith, meekness, temperance" (Gal. 5:22-24).

Let's examine more closely some of this beautiful clothing which should adorn the soul.

I. FAITH is the basis for all other virtues.

What is faith? It is believing what God says — believing his commands enough to obey them, believing his warnings enough to heed them, and believing his promises enough to be comforted and sustained by them. Faith can come only through a knowledge of God's word (Rom. 10:17).

Without this faith in God, man is like a ship without rudder or anchor, tossed mercilessly and aimlessly upon the sea of life. Dr. David Seabury, a clinical psychologist, said: "I have never been able to bring a man back to sanity and right thinking until I have brought him first to a faith in God."

Faith gives one power to be more than a conqueror (Rom. 8:37). The obstacles last but for a time; the victory extends into eternity — victory over sin, sorrow, fear, persecution, heartaches. These can be overcome, and "joy cometh in the morning" (Psalms 30:5).

All conduct springs from what one believes. Faith is the root; conduct is the fruit. For example: one who has no belief in an eternal existence will surely make little effort toward righteousness. A young convict was asked if he felt any remorse for his past deeds. His reply was: "Why should I? I don't believe in God or eternity, so why shouldn't I do as I please here?" Disbelieving, or even doubting, the absolute certainty of God's word will lead to a disintegration of the moral fiber of an individual or a nation; for it leaves no incentive toward righteousness and no restraint from evil. Beliefs control deeds, and deeds determine destinies. Yes, what one believes is of paramount importance.

II. COURAGE stems from faith.

"I had fainted, unless I had believed" said the Psalmist (Psalms 27:13). "Be of good courage, and he shall strengthen your heart, all ye that hope in the Lord" (Psalms 31:24).

There is no place for the faint-hearted in God's service. Real courage is required to stand in the face of ridicule, return good for evil, love enemies, and endure trials and sorrows.

> Of all the virtues in the world,
> Two things stand like stone —
> Kindness in another's troubles,
> And courage in your own.

Courage is contagious. Barak said to Deborah, "If you will go with me, I will go" (Judges 4:8). Courage flowed from Deborah through Barak and on to 10,000 soldiers to bring victory to God's people. We need to be courageous, not only for our own good, but also for the sake of others. The courage of one has many times rallied a cause from seeming defeat to victory.

III. PEACE of mind and security of spirit are the keenest longings ever experienced.

These longings of the soul must be satisfied, not by a stifling of the conscience, but *through a compliance with God's word.* This brings reconciliation with both God and fellowman, and being at variance with either will produce an indescribable disquietude. It is impossible to enjoy real peace without being at war — at war with all that is evil and sinful.

2. *Those who possess "the peace of God which passeth all understanding"* (Phil. 4:7) can help others to find it. Christ could say, "My peace I leave with you," because he was at peace himself — a peace unrelated to outside circumstances. In the midst of a turbulent world, peace can be found only beneath the stormy surface. It is comparable to the depths of the ocean which remain undisturbed by surface storms no matter how frequent or violent they rage. Such peace is priceless. One may have wealth, health, power, friends, and loved ones — but without peace of mind he is poor and wretched indeed.

IV. GENTLENESS AND KINDNESS are such beautifying qualities, yet all too rare.

Abigail exemplified gentleness. Even though she was married to a churlish drunkard, she refused to become imbittered or harsh in dealing with others. Her gentle appeal to David is one of the most touching and effective speeches recorded in the Scriptures (I Sam. 25:3-38).

"In her tongue is the law of kindness" (Prov. 31:26). "That which maketh a man to be desired is his kindness" (Prov. 19:22, A.S.V.) It has been said that kindness is the oil in the cogs of life's machinery.

V. HUMILITY is actually a realization of our dependence upon God and fellowman and the proper relationship we sustain to each. The truly great are humble.

"The ornament of a meek and quiet spirit, which is in the sight of God of great price" (I Peter 3:4-6). A reading of the entire passage shows that this desirable ornament caused women of old to obey their husbands, realizing their God-given relationship.

Humility is necessary in becoming a Christian, for one must completely submit his will to the will of God. When this is done, then God "will beautify the meek with salvation" (Psalms 149:4). Those too proud to admit this dependence upon God will forever remain outside his family.

VI. PATIENCE will bless us and all who associate with us.

Patience with erring Christians. "Ye which are spiritual

restore such a one" (Gal. 6:1). More patience by mature Christians could have retrieved many.

Patience in efforts to achieve. James Watt, inventor of the steam engine, said: "The world has heard of my success, but only my nearest neighbors knew of my repeated failures." Failure is often the vestibule to success.

Patience in hardships. Reverses may be blessings, for they help to strengthen the soul. "Tribulation worketh patience" (Rom. 5:3). God may be helping us to learn patience. A woman once said: "I prayed for patience, and God sent me a stupid servant girl to help me develop it." "How poor are they that have not patience! What wound did ever heal but by degrees?" —Shakespeare.

Some even become impatient with God because he does not punish evil-doers as quickly as they would like (Psalms 37:7-9).

One of the greatest needs for patience is in meeting the problems that one must face in *the everyday affairs of life.* Without this needed and pleasant characteristic, one is sure to be overcome with irritation. This blights an otherwise beautiful character. One of the reasons that everything seems to run so smoothly for some people is that they have acquired patience.

VII. FAIRNESS in thought, in action, in dealing with others and with God, is one form of honesty.

Two women met for the first time in many years. Anxious to catch up on all the news, Mrs. A. said: "And tell me about your children. How is Mary?" Mrs. B. replied: "Oh, she is getting along wonderfully. She is married to the dearest man in the world. He gets up every morning and prepares his own breakfast, goes to work and never wakes Mary at all. Then in the evenings, he helps with dishes and does so many things around the house. Oh, he's such a sweet man." "How nice," said Mrs. A; "and how is your son John getting along?" "It makes me sad just to think of John," responded Mrs. B. "John is married too, but he has such a hard time. You know, he has to get up every morning and manage for his own breakfast while the lazy wife of his sleeps. Then he works hard all day making a living for her and the children; and when he comes home she still expects him to help with the dishes and do all sorts of things that she should have been doing all day. John has such a hard time."

This type of unfair thinking is at the root of so much criticism, dissension, and unrest.

A complete sense of fairness toward others can best be achieved by projecting ourselves into their place and visualizing how we would want to be treated (Matt. 7:12).

VIII. WISDOM is a priceless asset in all phases of life.

The person of wisdom and good judgment will become a citadel of strength for many others. Deborah's wisdom made her counsel invaluable, and all Israel found their way to her judgment seat underneath the palm tree (Judges 4:5). The world beats a pathway to the door of those who are really wise.

How does wisdom come? "The fear of the Lord is the beginning of wisdom; a good understanding have all they that do his commandments" (Psalms 111:10). The ability to size up any problem and find its solution from the truths of God is an attribute valuable and much to be desired. This ability can be increased with effort and prayer (Jas. 1:5). We must strive to become "wise as serpents, and harmless as doves" (Matt. 10:16). How this world needs men and women with enough mature judgment and common sense to think straight and deduct sound conclusions.

IX. LOVE is the beautiful overcoat which should surround all other virtues, creating a picture of loveliness. "And above all these things put on love, which is the bond of perfectness" (Col. 3:14).

Poets, orators, and artists have sought to depict the strength and beauty of love, but *it may best be defined by examining the way it acts.* Love is that force which causes one to obey God (Jno. 14:21-23), and to do good to an enemy (Matt. 5:44). Read in I Corinthians 13:4-8 a description of the behavior of love — whether toward husband, wife, parents, children, friends, or enemies.

Love of the brethren is one of the tests of discipleship (Jno. 13:35). This God-like quality must pervade every phase of the Christian's life. "Love is precisely to the moral nature what the sun is to the earth." —Balzac.

EXERCISE

1. How can faith be increased? ....
   ....

2. Faith can be strong enough to enable one to be "more than ...."

3. "I had ...., unless I had believed."

4. What Bible woman is cited as one who was a source of courage for many others? ....

5. What did Solomon say would make "a man to be desired"? ....

6. What was the ornament specified by Peter? ....

7. God will "beautify the meek with ...." Why is meekness necessary before one can become a Christian? ....

8. Fairness toward others may best be achieved by following ....

9. "The fear of the Lord is the beginning of ...."

10. What is the lovely overcoat (the mink stole!) which should bind all other adornments of the heart together? ....

11. Love toward God causes one to .... him.

12. If one says he loves God but hates his brother he is a .... (I John 4:20).
13. "Be of good ... . and he shall .... your ...., all ye that hope in the Lord."
14. List the lovely robes for the heart mentioned in Galatians 5:22-24 ....
....

FOR THOUGHT OR DISCUSSION

1. Why does disbelief in the Bible lower moral standards? Are there fruits of such today?
2. Does humility demand that one be blind to his own abilities and accomplishments? Consider Paul's confidence expressed in Philippians 4:13; then give a definition of real humility.
3. Discuss the behavior of love as stated in I Corinthians 13:4-8.
4. How can peace of mind be attained even in the midst of the most trying circumstances?

V

Disposition Diseases

IT is not possible to over-emphasize the seriousness of sins of disposition. They are the sins of the heart, that part of us which will never die. If our hearts are diseased and warped by sin, what poor and mishapen things we will be to step into eternity.

Some have the mistaken idea that at death God will transform all our wicked ways and send us right on into heaven. Such is not true. As we die, so shall we spend eternity.

It is possible for women, by disposition and behavior, to win or fail to win others to the Lord (I Peter 3:1). Sins of disposition have caused many Christians to eclipse the saving light of the gospel. Our attitudes either verify or deny our relationship with Christ. A child once asked his mother: "Am I kin to Jesus on your side or on Daddy's side?" Our dispositions should reveal a close kinship with the Master. Let's consider some sins of the heart which mar spiritual beauty.

I. INGRATITUDE is a characteristic of the wicked (II Tim. 3:2); yet how many today are not grateful to God or man.

Shakespeare aptly expressed it: "Blow, blow, thou winter wind! Thou art not so unkind as man's ingratitude." How blessed is the child who is taught to be grateful.

Ingratitude toward God is most often *seen during times of prosperity,* as exemplified by the children of Israel (Deut. 31:20).

Unthankfulness is often *shown toward friends and family,* as Job experienced (Job 19:14-16).

The sincere expression of gratitude is *an admission that*

one is indebted to others, and pride keeps many from doing so. Remembering the many blessings received from God and fellowman should produce gratitude, but how short are our memories at times. Learn to say "thank you" freely to God, to friends, and to loved ones. It will enlarge your heart and bless you. Deep gratitude is one mark of true greatness.

II. SELFISHNESS is the root of so many other evils.

"Look not every man on his own things, but every man also on the things of others" (Phil. 2:4). A spirit of complete unselfishness was the golden thread which tied Ruth and Naomi together in such a sweet and harmonious way. It will help promote peace in any realm.

A little boy passed a basket of apples to his playmate, who took the biggest one. The boy chided: "You selfish thing; I thought you would take the little one and leave the big one for me." How like the motives that often prompt adults too.

III. STUBBORNNESS was punishable by death under the law of Moses (Deut. 21:18, 19).

This testifies to the seriousness of it. It springs from a refusal to recognize any authority but one's own will, and results in much domestic and church strife. Some are like the woman who said to her husband: "Well, all right, I'll admit I'm wrong, if you will admit that I am right."

IV. DISCONTENT is prevalent even among Christians.

One basis for discontent with many is their foolish efforts to be somebody they are not. Our materialistic age has increased the problem, for much discontent springs also from an overemphasis of *things,* a lop-sided sense of values. Wise and happy is one who learns early in life the lesson given by Christ: "For a man's life consisteth not in the abundance of the things which he possesseth" (Luke 12:15). An ancient proverb says: "Enough is as good as a feast."

> What matter will it be, O mortal man, when thou are dying,
> Whether on a throne or the bare earth thou are lying?
>
> —From the Persian

Contentment is produced, not by what is around us, but by

that which is within us. It comes from a realization of true values and a compliance with God's commands — contentment born, not of indifference or indolence, but from the assurance that "my God shall supply all your needs." This should serve as a divine tranquilizer. Think of the all-inclusiveness of this statement: "Godliness with contentment is great gain" (I Tim. 6:6). One who is godly and contented is truly rich!

V. PRIDE is one of the things hated by God (Prov. 6:16, 17). It is the basis of many related sins in the lives of Christians. Those who exalt themselves are riding high for a fall (Luke 14:11). Really, there is no place for pride. Surely the wicked have nothing of which to boast; and even the most godly are still only sinners who have been saved by the mercy of God.

Pride is completely contrary to the spirit of Christ. A lesson might be learned from the little boys who scrawled in childish print in their clubhouse this motto: "Nobody act big. Nobody act little. Everybody act medium."

> Humble we must be if to heaven we go;
> High is the roof there; but the gate is low.
> —Robert Herrick

VI. ENVY is one of the most prevalent and deadly evils.

Envy is the daughter of pride and the mother of hatred, vengeance, murder, and other sins which taint the soul with filthy slime. It crucified Christ, sold an innocent Joseph into bondage, and caused the godly David to have to flee as if he were a hunted animal from the insanely envious Saul. Let's consider some thoughts which should help conquer this sin.

It is a work of the flesh which can condemn the soul (Gal. 5:21).

It is an admission of a feeling of inferiority, directed most often against one's equals rather than against those admittedly superior in another field. For example: a woman is more likely to envy the accomplishments of her friends than she is to envy a Queen Elizabeth or some movie star.

God reasoned with Cain, whose envy led him to kill his brother: "If thou doest well, shalt thou not be accepted?"

(Gen. 4:7). But envy is unreasonable. Cain felt that he had suffered by comparison (I John 3:12), and he was obsessed with a desire to get rid of the object of his envy.

Two jay birds were once seen fighting over one elderberry while a whole bush of elderberries were ripe nearby. We should have more than "bird brains." There are enough "elderberries" to go around, if one is willing to put forth the effort to obtain them.

We should realize that *envy actually destroys its possessor*, being the "rottenness of the bones," a cancer, a viper which sucks the life blood from those who clasp it to their bosom. We have all seen logs going downstream caught on a rock, never reaching their destination. Many today are caught on the rock of envy and resentment — while the stream of life's good things passes them by.

The envious are doubly miserable — pained not only by their own troubles but also by the successes of others.

VII. HATRED AND MALICE are often born of envy.

Such a feeling causes one to be guilty of murder (I John 2:9-11; I John 3:15). A feeling of hatred in time gives birth to a spirit of vengeance and retaliation. Many years ago in a fashionable district in Brooklyn a woman developed such intense dislike for her neighbor that she had a fourteen-foot wall built around her property. Before long, her own flowers and shrubs withered and died from a lack of sunlight — while her neighbor's bloomed on in all their beauty. Vengeance is a boomerang which returns with more venom than it sends forth. Even the world loses respect for the spiteful person.

None can afford to pay the high cost of hating. How good was God to us when he commanded: "Avenge not yourselves. . . Vengeance is mine, I will repay" (Rom. 12:19). We can let the Lord take care of vengeance and save ourselves from being hardened, imbittered, and poisoned. Paul did this: "Alexander the coppersmith did me much evil: the Lord reward him according to his works" (II Tim. 4:14).

The following was written by an inmate in a Maryland penitentiary:

> Sowing the tares, when it might have been wheat;
> Sowing of malice, spite and deceit.
> We might have sown roses amid life's sad cares
> While we were so cruelly sowing the tares.

VIII. A SPIRIT OF UNFORGIVENESS cuts our own lifeline to heaven.

Receiving forgiveness from God is conditioned upon our willingness to forgive others (Matt. 6:14, 15). A minister once walked sixty miles to ask George Washington to pardon a man sentenced to death for treason. Washington refused. The minister explained: "I suppose I have not a worse enemy than the man who is about to die." This spirit of forgiveness so touched Washington that he relented and pardoned the man.

IX. A DOMINEERING SPIRIT is the age-old spirit of Jezebel.

By "steam roller" tactics she got her way, regardless of the consequences to others. She thought she knew all the answers. She was ready to give the orders, and heaven help those who violated them! She led her husband and three children into evil, miserable, and tragic lives. They would have fared better with no wife or mother at all. Modern "Jezebels" still live, bringing misery to all around them.

An interesting news item appeared in the paper recently, coming from Johnston, Iowa. It is reputed that Dr. Wade Smith, who is associated with a poultry company which sells 40,000,000 chickens yearly said: "We have discovered that every flock of hens has its dominating dowager and a special social rating for every one of its members. The most important hen lords it over all the others and terrifies them to such an extent that it interferes with their feeding and their laying. But that isn't the end of it. The second most important lady in the flock also puts the hex on hens who are beneath her in the social scale. And so on down to the last miserable chicken in the social register." The company is spending a considerable amount of money in an effort to correct the problem.

What unhappiness is wrought by people obsessed with the idea of becoming "the biggest hen in the pen" — whether in the home, church, or community.

EXERCISE

1. Will death change our dispositions? ....
2. What did Peter teach about disposition or behavior in winning others to Christ? ....
   ....
3. Which attribute is cited as outstanding in the sweet relationship enjoyed by Naomi and Ruth? ....
4. How bad did God regard stubbornness under the law of Moses? ....
5. Christ said that the more material things we have, the happier we will be (T or F).
6. "................ with .... is great gain."
7. Prove that God hates sins of disposition. ....
   ....
8. Cain hated Abel because ....
9. Name three Bible characters who suffered at the hands of envious persecutors: (1) .... (2) ....
   .... (3) ....
10. Envy is likened to the "................ of the bones."
11. In what two ways are envious people miserable? ....
    ....
12. "Whosoever hateth his brother is a ...."
13. Which verse proves that man should not take vengeance on those who wrong him? ....
14. Forgiveness from God can come only to those who practice .... toward others. Scripture: ....

FOR THOUGHT OR DISCUSSION

1. Can you think of some practical ways of teaching gratitude to children?
2. When Cain killed Abel, the object of his envy, did he eliminate his problems or did he bring upon himself more grievous ones?
3. Do you think God is going to admit into heaven the domineering personality who would want to start telling him how to manage heaven?
4. Are we acceptable in God's sight just as long as we don't *do* anything wrong, or can the sins of the heart condemn us?
5. Consider this statement from Dr. Paul Popenoe: "Of all the influences which play a part in the genesis of criminality, the mother's personality appeared to be the most fundamental."

VI

A Matter of Life and Death

WARS are started and wars are ended, not with bullets, but with words. It is hardly possible to evaluate fully the power of the tongue. Speech is an affair of the heart, an aspect of disposition so vital that it needs frequent study. Words are a definite index to the heart, for, "out of the abundance of the heart the mouth speaketh" (Matt. 12:34). Every word originates in the heart and broadcasts to the world the true condition of the inner being. We tell on ourselves. Others know what we are by what we say. We only deceive ourselves if we imagine it is otherwise.

I. "DEATH AND LIFE ARE IN THE POWER OF THE TONGUE" (Prov. 18:21).

A man once said to his son: "In talking, use as much caution as a carpenter: measure twice and saw once." *For our own good, we must learn to watch our words;* for "Whoso keepeth his mouth and his tongue, keepeth his soul from troubles" (Prov. 21:23).

It has been said that the best bridal admonition a mother can give her daughter is: "Daughter, bridle your tongue." Truly this is wise, for God says, "If any man offend not in word, the same is a perfect man, and able also to bridle the whole body." Read James 3:2-14. Though the tongue cannot be tamed, it must be controlled — just as some wild animals can never be domesticated, but they can be controlled so that they do no harm. We never outgrow the necessity of constantly watching the tongue lest it harm and destroy. It is never tamed to the extent that it can be given free range.

Sins of the tongue are so serious that *they can cause one's religion to be altogether in vain* (Jas. 1:26). The tongue can be a deadly poison destroying peace and happiness, as poison does the human body, for ourselves as well as for others (Jas. 3:8). Words can condemn one at the day of judgment: "For by thy words thou shalt be justified, and by thy words thou shalt be condemned" (Matt. 12:37). No wonder God said: "Death and life are in the power of the tongue."

II. SINS OF THE TONGUE.

Murmuring and complaining can become such a habit that nothing goes right. God says: "Do all things without murmurings and disputings" (Phil. 2:14). The murmuring children of Israel are cited as examples to warn against such (I Cor. 10:10). Constant complaining requires no talent whatsoever and serves only to develop an undesirable personality and annoy all who must listen to it.

Anger and uncontrolled temper. Angry words can sever some of life's sweetest bonds, but "a soft answer turneth away wrath" (Prov. 15:1). In the battle of New Orleans, Andrew Jackson stopped cannon balls of the British artillery with bales of cotton.

Anger is sometimes justifiable, but we must watch lest it lead us into sin: "Be ye angry, and sin not: let not the sun go down upon your wrath" (Eph. 4:26). He who cannot control himself cannot successfully guide others. "He that hath no rule over his own spirit is like a city that is broken down, and without walls" (Prov. 25:28).

Some people even boast: "I say everything I think" — not realizing that they are marking themselves as foolish. God says: "A fool uttereth all his mind" (Prov. 29:11). Silence is one virtue within the reach of everyone. It can be a priceless asset at times.

Contention and nagging. God gives very graphic descriptions of a contentious woman: like a constant dripping (Prov. 19:13; 27:15). A leaky faucet can drive one to distraction! And it is more pleasant to dwell in the wilderness than with such a woman (Prov. 21:19).

Delilah tried it on Samson. She pressed him daily until he was "vexed unto death" (Judges 16:16). She finally won her point. She got her way. But it brought to both unhappiness and then destruction.

Some are like the little girl who was asked if she could spell banana. She said, "Yes, I know how to spell it, but I don't know when to stop." The dictionary defines nagging as "constantly urging."

It is deplorable that this sin is found most often in the family circle; for the home should be a haven of rest, peace, and strength for all members of a family. Contentious wives are not only helping to fill divorce courts, but medical authorities say that such can be a contributing factor in the increase of early heart failures among men. A doctor warns: "To keep your husband alive, don't keep him in a stew." Surely many early deaths occur which are not the fault of either mate; but this doctor's statement does furnish food for thought. These principles also apply, of course, to contentious husbands or any other member of a family.

"Follow after the things which make for peace" is a command of God (Rom. 14:19). Contentious and angry words promote strife instead of peace and openly violate this commandment.

Impure speech. "Let no corrupt communication proceed out of your mouth" (Eph. 4:29). The influence of many Christians has been destroyed by telling that which sounded clever but not clean. The dirty story advertises the condition of the heart.

Surely profanity should also be out of the question for a Christian. Profanity is a light regard for sacred things. Taking God's name in vain (Ex. 20:7) is one form of it. "Out of the same mouth proceedeth blessing and cursing. My brethren, these things ought not so to be" (Jas. 3:10).

Lying has become so prevalent that in many circles one who practices absolute truthfulness is considered naive. But Satan is the father of all lies (John 8:44), and all liars will spend eternity with him (Rev. 21:8). A lying tongue is one of the things God hates (Prov. 6:16-19). Yet how many children learn from their parents to lie when it will further their own interests in some way.

You Can Be Beautiful

6. *Gossip* is forbidden by God: "Thou shalt not go up and down as a talebearer among thy people" (Lev. 19:16). Nevertheless, many otherwise good people can participate freely in destroying someone's good reputation and still seem to feel no remorse of conscience or guilt of sin. God spoke of some women as being "idle, wandering about from house to house; and not only idle, but tattlers also and busybodies, speaking things which they ought not" (I Tim. 5:13).

"How great a matter a little fire kindleth! And the tongue is a fire . . . and setteth on fire the course of nature; and it is set on fire of hell" (Jas. 3:5, 6). The church has its pyromaniacs who enjoy starting a little fire and then watching it grow into a great blaze.

"A talebearer revealeth secrets: but he that is of a faithful spirit concealeth the matter" (Prov. 11:13). Notice that it does not say: "A talebearer is one who tells lies." Many true things should not be repeated, and God condemns "tattlers . . . speaking things which they ought not." Some minds, like vultures, feast upon the most corrupt things to be found.

When we preface a statement with one of the following phrases, let's stop and search our hearts before proceeding: "Have you heard . . ." "Keep this to yourself, but. . ." "They tell me. . ." "I don't believe it's true, but. . ."

Gossip can wound hearts, destroy friendships, wreck homes, promote strife, and tear down the influence of the church in any community. It is contrary to every Christian principle and promotes nothing good whatsoever.

7. *Fault-finding* is regarded by many as a harmless American pastime, but such has always been condemned by God. He ridicules those who would dissect and analyze the faults of others while being guilty of sins so much more grievous (Matt. 7:3-5). The chronic fault-finder attempts to elevate himself by dwelling on the weaknesses of others; but we shall be judged, not by the mistakes of others, but by the perfect standard set forth in God's word. Adam used fifteen words to tell of Eve's sin, and only three words finally to admit his own. It is so much easier to see others' weaknesses.

Harsh and unkind words. "She openeth her mouth with wisdom; and in her tongue is the law of kindness" (Prov. 31:26). "Be ye kind one to another" (Eph. 4:32). Yet some seem to be unable to resist the acid retort. Remember that a lot of little digs will eventually bury love or friendship. And let's never be guilty of mistaking sarcasm for humor. A sarcastic remark is never funny, no matter how cleverly it is veiled. One who frequently jokes at the expense of another's feelings displays his own immaturity and sense of insecurity and inferiority. In an effort to elevate himself by stepping on someone else, he actually lowers himself.

III. THE TONGUE AS BEAUTIFUL "AS CHOICE SILVER."

"The tongue of the just is as choice silver" (Prov. 10:20). "A word fitly spoken is like apples of gold in pictures of silver" (Prov. 25:11).

If all the world were stricken dumb, what crimes and evil would cease. But think what good would also stop. Within the tongue lies the power to bless all mankind: to encourage the faint-hearted, teach the word of God, comfort the sick and sorrowing, spread cheer, impart wisdom, pray, and sing praises to God. *"Death and life are in the power of the tongue."*

> A careless word may kindle strife;
> A cruel word may wreck a life;
> A bitter word may hate instill;
> A brutal word may smite and kill.
>
> A gracious word may smooth the way;
> A joyous word may light the day;
> A timely word may lessen stress;
> A loving word may heal and bless.

—Author unknown

EXERCISE

1. Every word originates in the .... Scripture: ....

2. "........................ and .... are in the power of the tongue."

YOU CAN BE BEAUTIFUL   45

3. How does Solomon say that one can keep his soul from trouble? ....
4. What does James say about the religion of one who does not bridle his tongue? ....
5. Will our words be mentioned at the day of judgment? .... Scripture: ....
6. What example did Paul cite to teach that it is sinful to murmur and complain? ....
7. What does Solomon say will turn away wrath? ....
8. "A .... uttereth all his mind."
9. "The contentions of a wife are a ....,"
10. Who is the originator of all lies? ....
11. People who are idle are likely to become "............................ also and ...., speaking things which they ....,"
12. Name seven things the Lord hates: .... How many of these concern the tongue? ....
13. The book of Proverbs says that a worthy woman will speak words of .... and ....
14. The tongue of the just is compared to ....

FOR THOUGHT OR DISCUSSION

1. A light regard for sacred things is profanity. For instance, it is said that Esau profaned his birthright; that is, he had little regard for that which was sacred. If one holds in his heart the proper sacredness toward God, can he take God's name in vain? Have you ever heard anyone use the name of his mother in an oath? How can any Christian esteem the name of God less?
2. How did Delilah get her way? Such a method may gain a temporary victory, but it can also destroy love and respect. If so, is the victory worth the price paid for it?

"LORD, IS IT I?"

When Jesus announced to his beloved apostles that one of them would betray him, each apostle began to search his own heart and to ask: "Lord, is it I?" (Matt. 26:22). Each did not point a searching or accusing finger at the other, but rather began to inquire about his own condition.

The following is *a very personal questionnaire* based on the principles covered in the two preceding lessons. May each meditate upon the questions and ask, "Lord, is it I?"

1. Am I so critical that I see a person's weak points quicker than I do the good points?
2. Am I so sensitive that I make myself miserable by taking in a personal way everything that is said?
3. Am I so childish that everyone else has to handle me with caution to keep me from getting mad and causing trouble?
4. Am I adult enough to accept a disappointment and adjust myself to it without feeling mistreated and making everyone around me miserable?
5. When a discourtesy is shown me, do I brood over it and determine to "get even"?
6. Am I always thinking that everyone else is out of step but me and that I could be happy if everybody else would just do right?
7. Can I control myself enough to watch my words, or do I half-way boast that I have a quick temper?

YOU CAN BE BEAUTIFUL 47

8. Do I hurt other people with my sharp and caustic remarks?
9. Do I have a habit of telling other people what to do?
10. Do I have bottled up inside me a feeling of hostility toward another?
11. Am I determined to have my way, regardless of what it may do to others?
12. Am I ever guilty of making sarcastic remarks about the accomplishments or successes of another?
13. Do I repeat that which should be kept secret and then excuse myself by saying, "But it's the truth"?
14. Can I be completely trusted with confidences?
15. When the good reputation of another is being undermined, do I participate?
16. Do I laugh at and encourage the telling of unclean jokes or stories?
17. When I realize that I am wrong, am I big enough to admit it; or do I still try to justify myself by trying to blame someone else for my conduct?
18. Do I "follow after the things which make for peace," or do my words and conduct promote strife?
19. Do I have too much pride to show real gratitude toward God and my fellowman?
20. Though it may be easy for me to "weep with them that weep," do I obey the other part of the verse which commands me to "rejoice with them that do rejoice"?
21. Do I attempt to white-wash my own sins by constantly pointing out the faults of others?
22. Do I bring unhappiness to myself and to others by frequent complaining?
23. Are others lifted up and made better by their association with me?
24. Am I willing to face my own weaknesses and admit them?
25. Do I ask God to help me overcome specific sins and to grow as a Christian?

VII

For Daily Application

GOD'S beauty formula includes many things. We could make a long list of Scriptures which should be observed each day. However, we are condensing a number of principles by citing only two Scriptures which, if observed daily, will help immeasurably toward spiritual improvement: (1) "Seek ye first the kingdom of God and his righteousness" (Matt. 6:33); and (2) "Study to be quiet, to do your own business, and to work with your own hands" (I Thess. 4:11).

It would be good for every Christian woman to attach these two Scriptures to some prominent place where she can meditate on them daily; for instance, over her mirror or above her kitchen sink. Using these as daily guides will help to make so many decisions.

I. "SEEK YE FIRST THE KINGDOM OF GOD AND HIS RIGHTEOUSNESS" (Matt. 6:33).

All of us live in two realms, the physical and the spiritual, and we have responsibilities in both. The major lesson taught in the tender story of Mary and Martha is the necessity of choosing "the good part" when a conflict arises in these two areas of responsibility (Luke 10:42). Christ rebuked Martha, not for household diligence, but for placing secondary matters above the more important values. This problem and its attendant decisions must be faced daily. Many people spend a lifetime majoring in minors, because they do not make the proper choices.

God must come first. "Thou shalt love the Lord thy God with all thy heart, and with all thy soul, and with all thy mind" (Matt. 22:37) — above family, friends, profession, social life, and everything else — but loving God first gives one the capacity to love others with more depth and tenderness than would otherwise be possible. On the other hand, giving only a part of self to the Lord keeps one torn and disquieted within.

Seeking the kingdom of God first will lead us to make the following decisions daily:

(1) *Church attendance.* When God comes first, it is unthinkable that household chores, yard work, company, recreation, or anything else should keep one from the place of worship. That decision is already made and requires not a second thought. Yet even the church has some "First Day Absentists." "Not forsaking the assembling of ourselves together" (Heb. 10:25) is a command given for our good. British sailors of old had a saying: "The seas are so great, our boats so small." The Christian who sincerely participates in worship is strengthened for future voyages on the sea of life. Realizing this need for strength will prompt us not to forsake any of the assemblies of God's people.

Thoughts such as these have helped to lead the feet of many toward the house of worship. Tell yourself: "Christ has promised to be there. I need the association of Christian people. I need spiritual food. It is a test of my love for God, and a love too weak to take me to worship is too weak to take me to heaven. My influence must be Christian. God has commanded worship for my own good to help me go to heaven."

(2) *Bible study at home.* If time is allotted for television, newspapers, and countless other things, but never for a study of God's word, will we not have to admit a violation of Matthew 6:33? It is impossible to be neutral. A failure to study and teach God's word at home speaks eloquently to others that we actually believe this: "God's word is not very important; we don't really have to follow it; the things of the world are more valuable than our souls." God commanded the Israelites to teach his word diligently to their children (Deut. 6:6-9). He also commands that such be done today (Eph. 6:4).

(3) *Prayer.* "The prayer of a righteous man availeth much" (Jas. 5:16). If we do not feel a need and desire to talk to God now, why would we want or expect to spend eternity with him? Prayer comes easily and naturally for those who put God first

in their lives. At any time, a Christian can draw upon this mighty source of strength, even silently in the midst of any circumstances.

The first recorded prayer in the Bible is that of a father in behalf of his son: "O that Ishmael may live before thee." The memory of praying parents serves as a mighty fortress to children in time of temptation.

> When father prays he doesn't use
> The words the preacher does;
> There's different things for different days,
> But mostly it's for us.
>
> I can't remember all of it,
> I'm little yet, you see;
> But one thing I cannot forget,
> My father prays for me.

(4) *The use of time and talents.* We must some day account for the use of our talents (Matt. 25:14-30). Anyone who can work in P.T.A., Dad's Club, Girl Scouts, make a dress, follow a recipe, or discuss current events certainly has talent that can be used for the Lord. A Christian mother who was active in school work was asked to teach a Bible class. She said: "I have never taught; but if I can be a room mother at school, I can teach a Bible class. If time does not permit both duties, I shall give up my school work." No wonder she has become an outstanding Bible teacher!

Time is sacred, because time is life. We can see the wisdom of the divine admonition to redeem the time (Eph. 5:16). Yes, the Lord holds priority on our time and talent.

(5) Following Matthew 6:33 will also *regulate our giving.* Scriptural giving is a natural consequence if one seeks first the kingdom of God. Our hearts will be where our treasure is (Matt. 6:21) — and our treasure will be invested where our heart is.

(6) *Decisions concerning social and recreational activities* should also be controlled by this principle. Social activities should be to life what the dessert is to the meal — not the whole menu. A diet unbalanced with too much dessert is weakening and sickening to the body. Likewise, a life unbalanced with too much social activity sickens and enfeebles the soul. Chris-

tians must constantly be on guard to prevent the whirl of social activities from relegating spiritual duties to second place.

The promised reward. If man will "seek ye first the kingdom of God," then the Lord has promised: "all these things shall be added unto you." It is conditional. God has promised to provide material needs — but only if we have placed spiritual things first.

II. "STUDY TO BE QUIET, AND TO DO YOUR OWN BUSINESS, AND TO WORK WITH YOUR OWN HANDS" (I Thess. 4:11).

This Scripture contains three forceful commands:

"Study to be quiet." How many woes come from too much talking! We usually have more cause to regret words than silences. ' The simple, silent, selfless man is worth a world of tonguesters" — Alfred Tennyson. Our preceding lesson shows the importance of thinking before speaking.

"To do your own business." Think what gossip, strife, and unrest would be prevented if this were obeyed. In every realm — home, church, school, business, and nation — so much heartache and trouble exists because some persist in attending to the business of others. "Your own business" — not everybody else's business. Diligence in discharging our own responsibilities will leave no time to care for the business of others. Our own work will take a lifetime.

"Work with your own hands." Work is God-ordained, a blessing for mankind, though we live in an age which regards the ability to get out of work as one mark of intelligence. This attitude has even invaded the church.

(1) *Think of the blessings of work.* Labor not only blesses others, but also rewards the worker. For instance:

There is the joy of accomplishment, without which no one can be happy. An idle, aimless existence brings nothing but misery and emptiness.

Work helps keep one out of trouble (I Tim. 5:13). Having busy hands is one of the most effective antidotes against being a busybody.

It helps to prevent over-sensitiveness. For example: when a little dog is ignored, he resents it; but when he is busy chasing a rabbit, he doesn't care whether he is noticed or not. Persons intent upon worthwhile projects seldom suffer the pangs felt by the super-sensitive. Their attention is centered upon something more important than seeming slights.

Woman's sweetest epithet was given in Proverbs 31:10 (A. S. V.): "a worthy woman." No appellation can be more significant. However, we learn from the chapter that such worthiness requires hard work; and it must be done willingly, with the right attitude and disposition, not regarding herself as a martyr or slave (Prov. 31:13). But look how sweet are the rewards: "Her children arise up, and call her blessed; her husband also, and he praiseth her. Many daughters have done virtuously, but thou excellest them all" (Prov. 31:28, 29). How much is it worth for your husband to say: "You're the greatest girl of them all"? Idleness and slothfulness do not evoke such praise.

(2) *Slothfulness has always been condemned by God,* as already cited in I Tim. 5:13. The godly woman "eateth not the bread of idleness" (Prov. 31:27). "If any would not work, neither should he eat" (II Thess. 3:10). However, the devil not only tempts us to be lazy, but he even helps to find an excuse for it. "The slothful man saith, there is a lion without, I shall be slain in the streets" (Prov. 22:13). What a ridiculous excuse! Yet it is no more so than some used today.

(3) *Thinking Christians will be diligent;* for life is so short, time is so precious, and there is so much to be done. "The slothful man roasteth not that which he took in hunting" (Prov. 12:27). Uncooked meat! Slothfulness can also leave houses unkept, meals unprepared, visits unmade, and souls untaught.

(4) *Many industrious women* try to shield their children from work, not realizing that one of the greatest favors which can be bestowed upon any child is the lesson of industry. It will bless him all the days of his life. An educator who counsels students in a state university stated that one of the most alarming traits of many young people is their "freeloading concept of life," an idea that the world owes them a living. Some-

You Can Be Beautiful

one has suggested that the following would be a good philosophy of life:

> Now I get me up to work;
> I pray the Lord I will not shirk.
> If I should die before the night,
> I pray the Lord my work's all right.

EXERCISE

1. List the two Scriptures suggested as guides for daily living.
   ....
   ....
2. We must love God with "all thy ...., and with all thy ...., and with all thy ...."
3. Do Christ's words to Martha mean that it is wrong to be a good housekeeper? ....
4. "The .... of a righteous man availeth ...."
5. Can parents bring up their children "in the nurture and admonition of the Lord" without teaching them God's word? .... Can this responsibility be discharged solely by taking them to Bible study on Sunday?
6. "And thou shalt .... them .... unto thy children, and shalt .... of them when thou sittest in thine house, and when thou walkest by the way, and when thou liest down, and when thou risest up." Scripture: ....
7. If God is not placed first by parents, are children likely to regard divine commandments as important? ....
8. Give the Scripture citation found in the lesson which proves that God regards laziness as wickedness. ....

9. Should we feed lazy people who are unwilling to work? .... Scripture: ....

10. Jesus said: "My Father .... hitherto, and I ...." (Jno. 5:17).

11. Among the rewards of the worthy woman: "her children ... call her ....," and her husband "............ .... her."

FOR THOUGHT OR DISCUSSION

1. Try to visualize what changes might be made in your daily life if all decisions were controlled by Matthew 6:33.

2. If we stay at home on Sunday night or Wednesday night to look at TV, have we failed to put spiritual things first?

3. When we are invited to social events which conflict with the time of worship services, what must the decision be?

4. Though recreation is good, can a day on the lake be substituted for worship? Or is it a sin to forsake the assembly of the church?

5. If Christians are busy discharging their own responsibilities, will they have time to try to attend to the business of the elders, preacher, or others?

6. Do your children know that you pray for them? Have they ever heard you?

7. Comment upon the difference between working of necessity and working willingly.

8. To determine what is actually the center of your life, make this test. When you are alone and your mind has free range, on what one thing does it most often center?

VIII

"Unspotted From the World"

AMERICA seems to find moral sins hilariously funny. So did Babylon. So did Rome. But moral decay always leads to political decay, and political decay brings national destruction. History should be sufficient warning to our nation, but today sin is held up as the great attraction of the age. Note the movie ads in your daily paper; the appeal is measured by the degree of sin portrayed.

What is funny about open immorality, broken homes, orphaned children, crowded hospitals, murderous highways, or the world's record in juvenile delinquency? Statistics show that each year in our nation deaths by violence almost equal the number of deaths by disease. Such is the magnitude of the fruits of sin.

Yet sin is so prevalent that many have been led to believe that they must engage in certain practices to be socially acceptable. No longer is an evil-doer frowned upon by society and considered to be different; now it is the righteous person who is generally thought to be out of step or just a little peculiar.

I. THE CHRISTIAN IS TO REMAIN UNSTAINED BY THE WORLD (Jas. 1:27).

After our souls have been cleansed by the blood of Christ, *we must "come ye out from among them, and be ye separate"* (II Cor. 6:17). "Be not conformed to this world" (Rom. 12:2). Children of God are to keep their souls unstained, "not having spot, or wrinkle, or any such thing," in order to be ready to enter eternity at any time (Eph. 5:27).

Such can be done, even against seemingly insurmountable odds. Joseph did. Noah's sons did. Would you not like to visit with Mr. and Mrs. Noah and ask them how they instilled within their sons strength enough to remain godly in the midst of unparalleled wickedness?

II. WHY DOES GOD WANT US TO LIVE FREE FROM WORLDLINESS?

Is it because he is a stern "kill joy" who does not want us to have a good time? Not at all. It is the very opposite. He loves us and wants us to be happy, and he knows what is necessary for happiness. He understands the following:

Sin always brings sorrow. Numerous examples, both Biblical and secular, testify to such. Adam learned that one of the first-fruits of sin is fear: "I was afraid," he said (Gen. 3:9, 10). The sinful are "utterly consumed with terrors" (Psalms 73:19). Satan can tempt one to sin and can even help furnish an excuse for sinning; but he is powerless to make a sinner happy in his sins. The treachery of sin lies in its deceitfulness. Byron, who surely tried all this world had to offer, concluded: "There's not a joy the world can give like that it takes away."

No sin can enter heaven (Rev. 21:27). God wants us to enjoy the bliss of heaven, so he commands us to put away all kinds of sin. Worldliness is one kind of sin.

Reaping what we have sown is an unalterable law of God (Gal. 6:7, 8; Job 4:8). This law, which operates in both the natural and spiritual realms, was set in order for man's good; but we can use it to our own destruction. God loves us too much to want us to reap the bitter dregs of a life of worldliness — but the reaping will surely follow the sowing. "For they have sown the wind, and they shall reap the whirlwind" (Hos. 8:7). What a pitiful and disappointing harvest! Byron further states:

> The thorns which I have reap'd are of the tree
> I planted; they have torn me, and I bleed.
> I should have known what fruit would spring from such a seed.

Worldliness is folly, the spirit of the child who lives only for the present hour regardless of the dangers of tomorrow, as Esau did. Belshazzar enjoyed his dainties and ignored the handwriting on the wall, but he wasn't smart to do so. "Fools make a mock at sin" (Prov. 14:9), but "a wise man feareth, and departeth from evil" (Prov. 14:16). It's smart to be good. It's foolish to do otherwise.

Worldliness destroys spirituality; and when spirituality is destroyed, the soul is lost. It is truly a bad bargain to purchase a few fleeting pleasures of sin at the cost of spirituality; for "the world passeth away, and the lust thereof," and then the soul is left desolate and unprepared for eternity.

III. HOW CAN WORLDLY ACTIVITIES BE DEFINED?

Satan is constantly trying to convince Christians that there is no harm in engaging in worldly practices just a little; thus, it becomes easy for some to believe that everything is all right. Shakespeare said: "There is no vice so simple but assumes some mark of virtue in his outward parts."

The question is often asked: "Then how can one know which practices must be avoided?" Surely God gives the standard of measurement.

That which destroys the body is sinful; for the body is sacred, the temple of the Holy Spirit (I Cor. 3:16, 17; 6:19, 20).

Any practice which destroys one's appetite for spiritual things is wrong. Love for God and love for the world cannot dwell in the same heart (I John 2:15-17). Many Christians, young and old, have gradually begun practices which seemed harmless, only to wake up later and find that they no longer loved and enjoyed spiritual things as they once did. Church attendance, Bible reading, association with spiritual people — all these had become dull and unappealing. The subtle and beguiling work of Satan had taken its deadly toll.

Any activity which leads one into sin must be shunned. Make the foresight test. Remember: when you pick up one end of a stick, you also pick up the other end. If a poisonous viper is on one end, neither end is harmless! Thus, one must examine the fruits and consequences of any practice to determine whether it is harmless.

Activities which destroy a Christian's influence and keep him from being "the light of the world" are wrong (Matt. 5: 14-16

Those things which have the "appearance of evil" must be avoided (II Thess. 5:22).

Specific sins mentioned in God's word are wrong beyond question, and many are definitely mentioned.

IV. MEASURING BY THE DIVINE STANDARD.

In the light of the foregoing principles, what worldly stains should the Christian avoid?

Sinful thoughts must be banished, "For out of the heart proceed evil thoughts, murders, adulteries, fornications, thefts, false witness, blasphemies" (Matt. 15:19). "As a man thinketh in his heart, so is he" (Prov. 23:7). Thoughts are affected also by what one sees and hears. Therefore, destructive movies, hurtful television, filthy literature, even degrading conversation, must be shunned. Read Philippians 4:8.

Worldly and sinful language is but an evidence of that which is in the heart (Matt. 12:34). Many Christians have dimmed their light and destroyed the influence of the Lord's church by a dirty story or a profane oath. All who would be beautiful to God must keep themselves free from this stain.

"Lasciviousness, revellings, and such like" are forbidden by the Lord (Gal. 5:21). Surely an honest appraisal of modern dancing will convince one that it is one thing included in this classification. Multitudes can testify to the destructive and heart-breaking fruit of the modern dance. Many educators, doctors, and social workers regard it as one of the gravest menaces facing our nation.

Drunkenness has become a national curse. It brings nothing but heartache to the guilty (Prov. 23:29-32), and to others also. Of course, the eternal consequences are worse, for drunkenness will keep one out of heaven (Gal. 5:21). The history of King Alcohol through the centuries has shown his power to destroy homes, happiness, influence, lives, and souls. Even in the nation of India, which we regard as heathen, all alcoholic beverages have been banned from state functions. This act, in contrast with our nominally Christian nation, should cause us to hang our heads in shame.

You Can Be Beautiful

Immodest dress should not characterize godly women; for the Lord admonishes: "In like manner, that women adorn themselves in modest apparel" (I Tim. 2:9). You remember that God clothed Adam and Eve (Gen. 3:21), teaching that all persons past the state of complete innocence should be clothed. A Christian mother wrote a most timely article called: "Live Bait for the Devil's Hook," emphasizing not only the sinfulness but also the peril involved in allowing girls to wear some of the modern scanty clothing.

The sins of the flesh catalogued in Galatians 5:19 — adultery, fornications, uncleanness, lasciviousness — can be more easily shunned by those who refuse to participate in some of the practices just discussed.

"As a jewel of gold in a swine's snout, so is a fair woman which is without discretion" (Prov. 11:22). God also speaks of "silly women" (II Tim. 3:6) and his eternal word warns against the "Delilahs" and "Bathshebas" of every age. Surely there can be no real beauty of soul apart from purity; and God has set this standard for men, women, boys, and girls alike.

Other sins may be recognized and avoided as we measure each by the standard given in the preceding section. One mark of Christian growth and maturity is the ability to "discern both good and evil" (Heb. 5:14). Such an admonition affirms that some things are evil and that the Christian must learn to recognize them and avoid them.

EXERCISE

1. Christians are to keep themselves "_____ from the world."
2. Adam soon learned that sin brings _____.
3. "Be not deceived; God is not mocked: for whatsoever a man _____ that shall he also _____ For he that soweth to the _____ shall of the flesh reap _____." Scripture: _____.

4. One who mocks at sin is considered by God to be a ....

5. "What! know ye not that your .... is the temple of the .... therefore glorify God in your .... and in your .... which are God's." Scripture: ....

6. Which Scripture forbids any practice which helps to destroy the body? ....

7. Is it possible to love the world and to love God too? .... Scripture: ....

8. "In like manner, that women adorn themselves in ....,"

9. Are all God's commandments given for our own good? .... Whom does it harm most when we disobey them? ....

10. "A wise man .... and .... from evil."

11. Job commented that those who plow .... and sow .... reap the ....

12. Give the six rules mentioned which help to determine the right or wrong of an activity:

   (1) ....
   (2) ....
   (3) ....
   (4) ....
   (5) ....
   (6) ....

FOR THOUGHT OR DISCUSSION

1. "Thou shalt not follow a .... to do ...." (Ex. 23:2). Does the fact that "everybody else does it" make any practice right? If we follow the majority, where will it lead us? See Matthew 7:13, 14.

2. After Adam and Eve sinned, they made for themselves clothing of .... Later they were clothed in animal skins by .... What do these incidents teach us?

3. Is it all right for the young to "sow their wild oats"? Can such sowing produce a happy harvest? Charles H. Spurgeon once commented: "When youth starts sowing wild oats, it is time for the father to get out the thrashing machine."

4. Does God give one moral standard for women and another for men?

5. Can a wrong or questionable practice be justified by pointing out that something else is just as bad?

IX
"Keep Me From Presumptuous Sins"

DAVID, who often asked divine aid in keeping his heart clear, prayed: "Keep back thy servant also from presumptuous sins" (Psalms 19:13). What are presumptuous sins? Anytime man sets aside the authority of God and presumes that his own way is just as good, he becomes guilty of presumptuous sin. Presumptuous is defined in the dictionary: "taking undue liberties; overbold."

Many are under the impression that immorality is the only sin and that clean living surely constitutes a lovely life in the Lord's sight. Surely such is necessary, but we are also given emphatic teachings on the gravity of violating God's positive religious commands. Since sin in any form or degree destroys spiritual beauty, our studies on how to be beautiful could not be complete without considering this aspect of sin.

Paraphrasing David's words, may each of us pray: "Lord, keep me from presumptuous sins." Let's consider some unchanging principles given by God.

I. LEARNING FROM THE LIVES OF OTHERS.

Moses committed a sin so serious that it barred him from the promised land. What was it? He smote the rock, when God had commanded him to speak to it (Num. 20:7-12). What was so bad about striking a rock? In so doing, Moses disregarded the authority of God and presumed to do as he pleased in the matter and to take unto himself credit that belonged to God. Moses passed many of his tests, but he failed this important one.

Though God had commanded animal sacrifice, *Cain presumed that something else would be just as good* (Gen. 4:2-5). If one does not respect the authority of the object of his worship, why engage in an act of worship? It avails nothing, and God rejected Cain's gift.

Nadab and Abihu were religious men, priests of God. When they offered strange fire which the Lord had not commanded, they were immediately consumed (Lev. 10:1, 2). Why such drastic punishment for a matter which seemed so small? It serves as testimony through all centuries that God's word must be respected.

Matthew 7:21-23 tells of some who will be condemned at the judgment even though they engaged in many acts of religion. Thus, one may perform some item of worship or service to God and sin in the very performance of it. As shown by these examples cited, it is not enough just to be religious. We must be religiously correct according to divine instructions. It does make a difference what we believe and what we do.

The sins mentioned in the four examples given above *involved no moral issue whatsoever.* These and other passages bear testimony to the fact that one may be morally good and still be guilty of sin — guilty of religious sin committed by adding to, or omitting, or altering in any way God's instructions to mankind.

II. WHY IS SUCH OBEDIENCE REQUIRED?

There is a sensible reason for every word and act of God. Why does he demand complete obedience? We may not know all the reasons, but we can see some basic principles involved.

He does so for our good. This life is a period of preparation. If we do not learn submission to the Father's will in this world, we will not be prepared for heaven where his authority reigns supreme. Obedience to all laws is for man's good. For example: we comply with traffic laws for our own protection. By obedience to the laws of health, we benefit ourselves. Likewise, obedience to spiritual laws is for man's own good.

The most fundamental principle in religion is this: **who has the authority to decide what man must do to go to heaven?**

God or man? A man preaching over the radio said: "I don't care what the Bible says about how to be saved; I can tell you a good way to get to heaven." Imagine such an attitude! Yet many who do not actually express it feel the same in their hearts. But surely the Creator with power to make man and to make heaven is the only one who can set the conditions of man's entrance into heaven. He is the gate-keeper at the portal of glory! How blasphemous of man to presume that he can go into heaven any way he pleases.

The principle of authority is under discussion in James 2:10: "For whosoever shall keep the whole law, and yet offend in one point, he is guilty of all." One who wilfully rejects God's authority on one point has actually rejected his authority on all points. For example: if your child obeys only those commands which please him, he has not obeyed you at all; for he would have omitted all your instructions if he had wished. So is our obedience to God. Those who follow the Bible commands which please them and ignore the ones that displease them have actually obeyed God in nothing. They have obeyed their own will.

III. GOD'S WILL IS GIVEN IN HIS WORD.

The only possible way for us to know what God wants us to do is through his word. It is complete and gives everything needed for the soul.

"All Scripture is given by the inspiration of God and is profitable for doctrine, for reproof, for correction, for instruction in righteousness; *that the man of God may be perfect, thoroughly furnished unto all good works*" (II Tim. 3:16, 17).

"According as his divine power *hath given unto us all things that pertain unto life and godliness*" (II Peter 1:3). Those who lived in the first century had all they needed to guide their souls to heaven. The same instructions can lead us to heaven. Nothing else can.

IV. SOME SERIOUS WARNINGS.

Since God is God, his word is authoritative. Those who would presume to alter it are, in effect, setting themselves up as wiser than God. Listen to these grave admonitions:

"Ye shall not add unto the word which I command you, neither shall ye diminish aught from it" (Deut. 4:2).

"But though we, or an angel from heaven, preach any other gospel unto you than that which we have preached unto you, let him be accursed" (Gal. 1:8, 9).

"Whosoever transgresseth, and abideth not in the doctrine of Christ, hath not God" (II John 9-11). We see that doctrine is much more important than many people have thought. The doctrine of Christ can be found only in the Bible. Doctrine not taught by Christ and the apostles in the first century — either by direct command, approved example, or necessary inference — must be rejected.

V. "THE COMMANDMENTS OF MEN."

In view of the foregoing Scriptures, we can better understand Matthew 15:9 which says: *"But in vain they do worship me, teaching for doctrines the commandments of men."* Christ also said: "Thus have ye made the commandment of God of none effect by your tradition" (Matt. 15:6). A human tradition is simply a practice of men which has been handed down from one generation to another. But commandments of men — whether they originated recently or centuries ago — can cause one's religion to be altogether in vain. Man must not presume to set aside the authority of God and substitute his own.

It is an undisputed fact that *many religious practices exist today which are not authorized in God's word.* We are forced to the conclusion that such originated with men rather than God. This realization should surely prompt us to examine every doctrine and practice to determine whether it came from God or men.

VI. MAKING THE TEST.

Understanding the foregoing principles, may we ask ourselves:

(1) *Who founded the church* of which I am a member? Was it founded by Christ or by some human being?

(2) *Is the religious name I wear* authorized by the word of God, or do I wear a name not found in the Bible?

(3) *Have I obeyed the same plan of salvation* set forth in the New Testament, which we studied in Lesson III? Do I believe in God and in Christ as the Son of God? Have I repented of my alien sins? Have I confessed before men the faith in my heart? Have I been baptized for the remission of sins, realizing that such is the scriptural purpose of baptism? Have I been baptized according to instructions given in the New Testament, by a burial in water?

(4) *Do I engage in the items of worship* set forth in God's word, or do I practice some things which were added by men?

Space forbids going fully into these and other aspects of our obedience to God. The major purpose of this lesson is to fix firmly in our minds the principle that a violation of God's positive religious commands is surely one kind of sin which can mar spiritual beauty and render us unfit to stand pure and blameless before the Great Judge. Wisdom demands that we carefully compare each item of our faith and practice to see if it is authorized by God. May we never be guilty of setting aside the will of God and following our own instead. May the attitude of our hearts always be: "Lord, keep me from presumptuous sins."

EXERCISE

1. What sin prevented Moses from entering the promised land?

    ....

2. "Nadab and Abihu... offered strange fire before the Lord, which he ...."

3. "Not everyone that saith unto me, ... shall enter into the kingdom of heaven; but he that .... the will of my .... which is in heaven."

4. "All Scripture is given by the .... of God and is profitable for ...., for ...., for

You Can Be Beautiful

..........., for instruction in ....: that the man of God may be ...., thoroughly furnished unto .... good works."

5. Give the three Scriptures cited which show that man must not alter God's law in any way: (1) .... (2) .... (3) ....

6. Following the commandments of men will cause one's worship to be in ....

7. Give two Scriptures to show that God gave his complete revelation in New Testament times: (1) .... (2) .... Does this positively prove that all so-called latter day revelations have come from men rather than God?

8. Keeping the whole law and offending in one point will: (1) be acceptable to God; (2) make one guilty of all; (3) be close enough to go to heaven. Number .... is correct.

9. Human tradition makes: (1) the commandment of God of none effect; (2) acceptable worship easier; (3) it easier to learn God's will. Number .... is correct.

10. He that abides not in the doctrine of Christ can still be saved (T or F).

FOR THOUGHT OR DISCUSSION

1. Did God tell Cain and Abel what kind of sacrifice to offer? Hebrews 11:4 says: "By .... Abel offered unto God a more excellent sacrifice than Cain." But how does faith come? See Romans 10:17. Therefore, we know that God had given them instructions concerning animal sacrifice.

2. Since the eating of fruit was not an immoral act, why was it sinful for Adam and Eve to eat the forbidden fruit?

3. When we start searching back into history and find that certain religious practices originated many centuries after the close of the New Testament period, what does this prove?

4. It would be good to consider the other principles set forth by David in Psalms 19:7-14.

X

Your Siamese Twins

OCCASIONALLY some women seem to resent their lot in life, stating emphatically: "It's a man's world; men have all the advantages." In this age-old discussion, a man once countered: "It's a woman's world. When a baby boy is born, people ask, 'How is the mother?' When a man is married, they exclaim: 'What a beautiful bride!' And when a man dies, they ask: 'How much did he leave her?'"

Nevertheless, it is good for men and women alike to be thankful for their respective advantages. God has showered abundant blessings upon all.

I. THE PRIVILEGE OF BEING A WOMAN.

Think of God's estimate of woman. Her creation was no haphazard after-thought. The Lord planned her to have tender emotional and physical qualities different from any other creature. She was the crowning act of all his creative power.

Think of Christ's estimate of woman; for he lifted her back up to a place of companionship with man, where God had originally placed her. Wherever Christianity has gone, women have been elevated. Before Christianity was introduced into the Fiji Islands, a man's widow was burned on his funeral pyre. Even in America, the Indians required their women to do the hardest work and to sleep in the coldest place in the wigwam. Women, of all people, should love Christ dearly. Without him, think what would be our plight both socially and spiritually.

Men respect women who are respectable. They want to be able to regard them as a source of strength and stability, pure, sweet, and very feminine. Listen to these men:

> There is no jewel in the world so valuable as a chaste and virtuous woman. —Cervantes.
>
> If there be any one whose power is in beauty, in purity, in goodness, it is a woman. —Henry Ward Beecher.
>
> A young man rarely gets a better vision of himself than that which is reflected from a true woman's eyes; for God himself sits behind them. —J. G. Holland.
>
> Earth's noblest thing, a woman perfected.
> —James Russell Lowell.
>
> Honor women! They strew celestial roses on the pathway of our terrestrial life. —Boiste.

II. THE PRIVILEGE OF BEING A CHRISTIAN.

Being a Christian is the most exalted privilege in the world. Think of some of the wonderful spiritual blessings: (1) past sins forgiven, (2) the assurance of being a part of the only indestructible thing in this world (Heb. 12:28), (3) promises of help and comfort in the midst of an uncertain and turbulent life, (4) the privilege of prayer, and (5) the hope of heaven.

Since noble womanhood *reaches the highest possibilities only through Christ,* how thankful we should be for the privilege of being Christian women.

III. EVERY PRIVILEGE HAS A SIAMESE TWIN CALLED RESPONSIBILITY.

PRIVILEGE—RESPONSIBILITY

This is true in every realm. For example: it is a privilege to be a parent, but the responsibility is ever present. The privilege of receiving a pay check carries with it the God-given duty of faithful work to the employer. Think of any privilege — to it you will find attached a responsibility.

Since the highest privilege is that of being a Christian, *to it are enjoined the gravest responsibilities.* Yet many seek to enjoy all the blessings of Christianity and ignore the attached duties. We may, like the ostrich, bury our heads and refuse to see the responsibilities; but they are still there and will face us at the judgment.

> I slept, and dreamed that life was Beauty;
> I woke, and found that life was Duty.
> Was thy dream then a shadowy lie?
> Toil on, poor heart, unceasingly;
> And thou shalt find thy dream to be
> A truth and noonday light to thee.
>
> —Ellen Sturgis Hooper

IV. RESPONSIBILITY THAT IS PERSONAL.

A realization of individual responsibility is one of the most urgent needs of the church today. So many want to go through life parking on the other fellow's nickel. Such will avail nothing at the judgment, for "every one of us shall give account of himself to God" (Rom. 14:12), and each life will be compared with what is written in God's word (Rev. 20:12). Each branch which does not bear fruit will be destroyed (John 15:2).

We are admonished: "Exercise thyself unto godliness" (I Tim. 4:7). "Exercise" — some effort must be exerted. "Thyself" — an individual matter; no one can discharge our duties for us: "Unto godliness" — this includes all God's instructions.

Thus, each Christian has a responsibility to: (1) develop a Christ-like personality, (2) be an influence for good at all times, (3) worship the Lord as he has commanded, (4) help promote the work of the church, and (5) teach others the truth.

V. RESPONSIBILITY THAT IS POWERFUL.

Think of the tremendous force which women exercise, either for good or evil. Recent tabulations show there are 2½ million more women voters than men, and that women spend 80c of every dollar spent. Concerning spiritual matters, think of the possibilities:

By word and example, mother is the child's first teacher. Though there are exceptions, the woman usually sets the spiritual tenor of the home. If she fails, how many souls may be led astray! How serious then should young mothers consider their spiritual responsibilities in the household.

The moral fiber of a nation is determined primarily by women. The rise and fall of nations may be traced by studying the women of the time. A nation can maintain a strength no greater than the homes that constitute it, and the home usually rises no higher than the ideals of the woman in it.

In each congregation much of the teaching must be done by women, both in classes and with individuals, for their schedules often permit time and opportunities not possible for men who must work.

If women are zealous in soul-winning, there is likely to be a spirit of evangelism throughout the entire church. If they are indifferent, the work of even the most consecrated men is hindered.

Women are often needed to help in benevolent works.

The spirit of hospitality, the use of homes in the Lord's work, is generally dependent upon the women.

> There's not a place in earth or heaven,
> There's not a task to mankind given,
> There's not a blessing or a woe,
> There's not a whispered yes or no,
> There's not a life, or death, or birth,
> That has a feather's weight of worth —
> Without a woman in it.

VI. WHICH WILL IT BE?

Yes, women wield a mighty impact — either for right or wrong, for victory or defeat. Many Bible examples testify to this fact:

A courageous Deborah led the nation of Israel to victory over God's enemies. The God-fearing Lydia and her household formed the nucleus from which the powerful church at Philippi developed.

On the other hand, the diabolical Jezebel was a fountainhead of evil and corruption which flowed through both Israel and Judah for centuries.

> O woman, perfect woman! What distraction
> Was meant to mankind when thou wast made a devil!
>   —John Fletcher

In every realm a woman can be either a source of strife

and evil, or she can be the one to pour oil upon troubled waters. In the home, she is either a part of the problem or a part of the solution. In the church, she is either a maker of peace or a promoter of strife.

VII. WHEN MUST THE BRAKES BE APPLIED?

Though the influence of women is everywhere felt, is there a limit to the use of her authority? Absolutely so. God has set limitations.

In the home the husband is her head, and she must be subject to him in all things unless such conflicts with her other duties to God (Eph. 5:22, 23; I Pet. 3:1-6). Thomas Fuller said: "She commandeth her husband, in any equal matter, by constant obeying him." The obedient wife gains far more than she loses!

Women are to work *under the oversight of the elders* of the church (Heb. 13:17). Thus, projects of ladies classes and all other church work of women should be under the elders' supervision.

Women are not to teach *in the public assembly of the church, nor to usurp authority over men* (I Cor. 14:34; I Tim. 2:11, 12). In spite of these Scriptures, a recent survey shows that seventy-two religious bodies in the United States now permit women equal authority with men, allowing them to preach and hold other offices. But God's word stands the same, and no human being has the right to nullify it and legislate a new policy.

Yes, the Lord has circumscribed for women places of service rather than positions of authority. In so doing, however, he has actually given women a formula for greatness: "He that is greatest among you shall be your servant." A respect for these divine limitations promotes happiness for women as well as for men.

EXERCISE

1. "............... .... of us shall give account of .... to God."
2. All will some day be judged by those things "written in the ...., according to their ...."
3. What will happen to the branch which does not bear fruit? ....
4. Cite at least two Bible women whose good influence is still remembered. ....
5. Cite a Bible example of a woman whose evil influence helped to corrupt two nations. ....
6. What is the greatest privilege which can be enjoyed in this world? ....
7. "Exercise .... unto ...."
8. "For the .... is the head of the ...."
9. "Obey them that have the rule over you, and submit yourselves: for they watch for your souls." This refers to obedience to the ....
10. "Let your women keep silence in the ....: for it is not permitted unto them to speak." Scripture: .... The assembly referred to is defined in the 23rd verse of the same chapter: "If therefore the .... be come together in one place."
11. This helps to clarify the teaching found in I Timothy 2: 11, 12. "But I suffer not a woman to teach, nor to usurp .... over the ...."

FOR THOUGHT OR DISCUSSION

1. If our girls understood that men like for women to look and act like women, do you think this would solve many of the problems of dress and conduct?
2. Is there any possible way to keep one's influence, either good or bad, from living on after he is gone?
3. Do you think our nation can ever be elevated morally unless women realize the necessity of doing so?
4. Is a woman to be subject to her husband even if he is not a Christian? Read I Peter 3:1-6. Was the husband referred to a Christian? What if he were to command her to disobey God? Read Acts 5:29.
5. We know that I Timothy 2:11, 12 does not forbid a woman ever to teach under any circumstances, for Titus 2:3, 4 specifies that women are to teach. Then what is the restriction placed upon the teaching done by women?
6. Does any individual or group have the authority to set aside the limitations which God prescribed for the authority of women?

XI

The Adorning of Sympathy

SYMPATHY, or compassion, means "to feel with" — the ability to put oneself in another's place and to feel as he feels. We should have sympathy for others, because God has first had compassion on us. In the parable of the Prodigal Son, God is represented by the father who "had compassion, and ran, and fell on his neck, and kissed him" (Luke 15:20). The parable of the unmerciful servant shows that even Christians fail many times to show compassion to others, forgetting that they themselves are wholly dependent upon God's mercy (Matt. 18:23-35).

Sympathy is an active quality, a spirit of kindness exemplified by a helping hand. This spirit may produce calloused hands from a soft heart. Too many in the world have the order in reverse — calloused hearts and soft hands. "Whatsoever ye would that men should do to you, do ye even so to them" will lead one to do as the good Samaritan (Luke 10:30-35). The church is filled with "priests" and "Levites" who excel in making a survey and reporting what should be done, but how few "Samaritans" there are to do the work.

I. SYMPATHY TOWARD THE SICK.

Sickness is an ever-present problem and always will be. Sooner or later each family is touched, regardless of station in life. What can be done to relieve the ill?

Administer to physical needs, if necessary. Modern facilities have lessened these needs; yet many still require assistance through long days and nights — someone to clean house, wash, iron, administer medicine, or prepare food.

Pray with them and for them, not only because God answers prayer, but because this manifestation of the faith and concern of fellow-Christians promotes courage in times of trial.

In many instances the only thing needed is *a visit to cheer and comfort*. Let's consider some practical suggestions gleaned from doctors and nurses, which should increase effectiveness in this field of service:

(1) Remember that the sick are weak and easily exhausted. Unless the patient is nearing recovery, the visit should be very brief. A doctor once said he wished relative to the Scripture, "And ye visited me," that the Lord had added the phrase, "and ye didn't stay long."

(2) Abide by requests for "No Visitors," and don't tell yourself: "That means everybody but me."

(3) Hold your voice down. Be cheerful but not boisterous. Over the door of one hospital is a sign: "If you can't smile, don't go in."

(4) Don't question the patient about his illness. If he mentions it, let him talk freely.

(5) Don't be tempted to prescribe your own remedies.

(6) Don't talk about others who have died with the same illness!

(7) In severe cases, don't enter the room at all unless needed or invited by the family.

(8) Don't touch the bed. A stream of bed-jostling visitors can drive a patient to distraction.

II. SYMPATHY TOWARD THE SORROWING.

"Jesus wept" (John 11:35). On another occasion, Jesus saw a woman sorrowing and "he had compassion on her" (Luke 7:13). This furnishes the answer to grief-stricken hearts who ask:

> Does Jesus care when I've said "good-by"
> To the dearest on earth to me,
> And my sad heart aches till it nearly breaks —
> Is it aught to Him? Does He see?
>
> —Frank E. Graeff

Christ-likeness includes the ability to "weep with them that weep" (Rom. 12:15). This will always be necessary, because there will always be sorrow until we reach that home where there is "no more death, neither sorrow, nor crying" (Rev. 21:4).

Some have said: "I am willing to help the bereaved, but I don't know what to say." Oftentimes it is needful to say little, if anything. Job's three friends came to comfort him and sat for seven days and nights before they said a word. Your presence bespeaks your love and interest. In making comments, however, the following points have proved helpful:

(1) Don't try to minimize one's loss. Losing a loved one is never easy, even though God's word gives so many consoling thoughts concerning the death of Christians.

(2) Don't try to stop their tears, for these are the safety valves of the heart.

(3) Don't try to divert their attention to trivialities. Rather, let them talk freely about the lost loved one, for talking helps relieve pent-up tensions. A preacher talking to a woman who had lost her husband said: "I didn't know your husband very well; tell me about him." She talked at length and when the preacher left she said: "I feel more relieved now than at any time since my husband's death."

(4) Almost without exception, those who lose loved ones are plagued by a guilt feeling as they recall things left undone and unsaid, a tendency to feel: "If we had only done this or that, perhaps death could have been postponed." An understanding that this is a common and natural reaction is reassuring to many.

(5) If death has taken a Christian, the consoling promises of God furnish the only real comfort. It is always good to pray with the bereaved.

(6) Words of comfort and deeds of thoughtfulness are sometimes more needed weeks or months after the death of a loved one, for it is then that most friends have gone their busy ways. Perhaps we can help to cushion the shock, until "time, like an ever-rolling stream, bears all our griefs away."

III. SYMPATHY TOWARD THOSE IN MATERIAL NEED.

This is one of the questions which will come up in our final examination (Matt. 25:31-46).

"Pure religion and undefiled before God and the Father is this, *to visit the fatherless and widows in their affliction*" (Jas. 1:27). In Acts 6:1-3 we read of the ministry of the church in behalf of needy widows in a day before social security, unemployment compensation, or city welfare. However, even then God placed restrictions upon those to be helped by the church. Christians are to care for the widows in their own family and "let not the church be charged" (I Tim. 5:3-16). We cannot disregard this command without being guilty of sin.

"As we have therefore opportunity, let us do good unto all men, especially unto them who are of the household of faith" (Gal. 6:10). God also places a restriction upon this: "that if any would not work, neither should he eat" (II Thess. 3:10). The Lord has never encouraged slothfulness, and instructs his children not to do so. Some need temporary financial assistance, but the vast majority are most in need of guidance to enable them to help themselves. To help someone to become self-sustaining is the best benevolence.

IV. SYMPATHY TOWARD THE LONELY.

The world is filled with those who need, not material assistance, but a *sympathetic friendliness.* Our efforts to cheer their hearts will cause our own troubles and despondency to dwindle.

The real *source of all strength and comfort* is God, "who giveth power to the faint... they shall run, and not be weary; and they shall walk, and not faint" (Isaiah 40:28-31); but fellow-Christians can help one to take hold of this power and to refresh his weary spirit.

> There are two kinds of people — you know them
> As you journey along life's track,
> The people who take your strength from you
> And others who put it all back.
>
> —Ralph Cushman

Even the smallest act of thoughtfulness usually thrills the heart of the elderly — a visit or telephone call, a brief pleasure ride, reading the Bible to them, a gift, a card, or a note of remembrance.

V. SYMPATHY TOWARD THE SINFUL.

Christ was condemned for eating with sinners and publicans, but they were *the ones most in need of him.* "They that be whole need not a physician, but they that are sick" (Matt. 9:12). Yet, some who claim to be followers of Christ have a Pharisaic spirit of condescension which reeks with a "holier than thou" flavor. Such has always been distasteful to God (Isaiah 65:5).

We must have sympathy toward *those who know not the truth.* Let's remember that if we had been reared and taught as they were, we would think and feel as they do. We should put ourselves in their places and teach them as tenderly as we would want to be treated. At no time is the following of the Golden Rule more important.

It is easy to become impatient with sinful Christians, but sympathetic helpfulness may "save a soul from death" (Jas. 5:19, 20). The attitude we must maintain in restoring the fallen is given (Gal. 6:1).

VI. SYMPATHY TOWARD THE JOYFUL.

Many who can easily "weep with them that weep" are unable to "rejoice with them that do rejoice" (Rom. 12:15). Yet, *this is a command* and one of the marks of a beautiful life.

Envy rises up within some hearts when others have cause for rejoicing. Such an attitude is positive proof of a lack of love, for "love envieth not." Love and envy cannot dwell together. When one walks in, the other walks out. True sympathy evokes not only weeping with the sorrowing but also rejoicing with the fortunate.

EXERCISE

1. To have sympathy means ....
2. Which Scripture teaches that we cannot expect mercy from God unless we have first shown compassion toward others?
   ....
3. Give two Scriptures which show that Jesus had compassion for those in sorrow. ....
4. List the things mentioned in Matthew 25:41-45 which will

come up at the judgment concerning our helping others.
....
....

5. "Pure religion and undefiled before God and the Father is this, to visit the .... and .... in their affliction."
6. Is it right to give material aid to those who are unwilling to work? .... Scripture: ....
7. Which Scripture is cited to show that God can assist those who are weary and discouraged? .... Read the entire passage.
8. God says that those who had a "holier than thou" attitude were like "............................. in my ...."
9. "Brethren, if a man be overtaken in a fault, ye which are spiritual, ... such a one in the spirit of ...., considering thyself, lest thou also be tempted."
10. Christians have a first obligation to help needy Christians rather than needy aliens (T or F). Scripture: ....
11. The shortest verse in the Bible is quoted in this lesson. What is it? ....
12. Pure religion is something: (1) you get; (2) you do; (3) you decree. Number .... is correct. Scripture: ....
13. Because of .... some people are unable to "rejoice with them that do rejoice."

FOR THOUGHT OR DISCUSSION

1. Since the Bible plainly states that Christians are to care for the widows in their own family and that the church is not to be charged with such care, discuss ways this can be done. Make a list of the homes and institutions in your area where such care can be purchased by those who cannot take widows into their own homes.
2. Are there any sure ways to recognize a sympathetic heart?

XII

"Awake Thou That Sleepest"

GOD admonishes Christians to wake up and says it is high time! (Eph. 5:14; Rom. 13:11). The only person who ever became famous while asleep was Rip Van Winkle, and even he didn't make a name for himself until he woke up! There's nothing pretty about a drowsy Christian. The Lord tells us to wake up. Why? Souls are dying, time is flying, and we need to be busy evangelizing the world. Christians have the power to do so, but just having the power is not sufficient. The most powerful machinery in the world is of no value until it is put into action.

We have discussed the tremendous power within Christian womanhood, but it will never be used much for the Lord until we are motivated, impelled from within. What are some of the motivating forces, the spark plugs, which can help to spark into action the unused force within Christians and to awaken sleepy saints to their responsibilities? A realization of the following principles would activate the whole church.

I. SOUL-WINNING IS BIG BUSINESS.

We can be partners with God in the greatest undertaking known to this world. No angel was ever allowed to teach the lost how to be saved, but man has been given this privilege. Surely this is a part of the lovely life, for God says: "How beautiful are the feet of them that preach the gospel of peace, and bring glad tidings of good things!" (Rom. 10:15).

Look around you. *Everything your eyes can see will some day be destroyed.* Only two things on earth will outlive this world and extend into eternity. One is the soul of man; the other is the word of God. Thus, the most vital task of life is to bring the soul of man into harmony with the word of God

— first, for ourselves; and secondly, to help teach others to do so.

II. THE MOST VALUABLE POSSESSION.

"*What shall it profit* a man if he shall gain the whole world and lose his own soul" (Mark 8:36, 37). Our materialistic age has caused many to lose sight of this. Standing atop the Empire State Building in New York, one can see an area of eighty miles in which live eighty million souls, each one worth more than all the material wealth the eye can view.

The Bible tells of a man who developed an intense desire to become a soul-winner — *after he got to hades* (Luke 16:27, 28). Then he understood the value of a soul, his and others, but it was too late. He woke up, but too late!

III. TAKING MEN ALIVE.

"And Jesus said unto Simon, Fear not: from henceforth, thou shalt catch men" (Luke 5:10). *"Catch men"* — this literally means "take men alive."

Every person you see is a never-dying soul. If we do not help to "take men alive" for God, then they must spend eternity with Satan. Surely this thought should impel us to be *fishers of men*.

IV. THE MAJOR WORK OF THE CHURCH.

The work of the church is two-fold.

The primary work of the church is to save souls.

(1) Teach the lost (Matt. 28:18-20). Christ left heaven, came to earth, spent a lifetime, and died to save the lost.

(2) Strengthen the saved (Matt. 28:18-20; Gal. 6:1). We must teach, then baptize, then teach some more. Restoring the fallen will "save a soul from death."

The secondary work of the church is to help the needy (Jas. 1:27). This is obviously secondary, for the soul is so much more valuable than the body. Relieving physical needs can serve, however, as one means toward saving souls.

V. THE URGENCY OF THE WORK.

Every minute there are approximately 180 souls departing this life, most of them unprepared (Matt. 7:13, 14). Working to save them is like working against the ticking of a time bomb. Time is running out for many at each tick of the clock.

Many would be receptive to the truth if someone would only care enough to teach them. *One of the saddest verses is:* "I looked on my right hand and beheld, but there was no man that would know me: refuge failed me: *no man cared for my soul*" (Psalms 142:4).

Do you remember the man at the pool of Bethesda who had no one to put him into the water (John 5:2-9)? Unhealed for the want of a friend. We would have helped him, we think. Yet how many are lost today because no one has cared enough to teach them. *Lost — for the want of a friend!* Is the task urgent? Immeasurably so!

Two small boys took the family clock apart and put it back together. During the night the father was awakened when the clock struck 117 times without stopping. "Sarah," he said excitedly to his wife, "you'd better get up! It's later than I ever knowed it to be!" This evokes a smile, and yet it's application is piercingly serious. It's later than we think. "Awake thou that sleepest!"

VI. WE MUST BE SOUL-WINNERS.

The command to teach the lost is enjoined upon each Christian (Matt. 28:18-20; Heb. 5:12; Phil. 2:15, 16). Christianity is like a course run in relays. The torch was lighted by God, Christ, and the Holy Spirit, who handed it to the apostles. They handed it to others, and someone handed it to us. Now we must pass it on. "Go ye into all the world and preach the gospel." Not everyone can go to Africa or China, but you daily move within your own little world — one that needs to be evangelized.

The blood of Christ is *the only remedy* for this sin-sick world. Trying to cure its ills with anything else is like trying to cure cancer with aspirin. Christians are the Great Physician's only helpers to take this eternal-life-giving remedy to the spiritually ill. If we fail, eternal death awaits them.

VII. WE CAN BE SOUL-WINNERS.

One of the basic needs of each person is for someone to convince him that he can do more than he thinks he can.

When Moses was asked to go to Egypt he said, "I can't." God said, "I will help you; and there will be others, such as Aaron, to help you." So Moses accepted the challenge to do something he had thought he could not do, and by so doing he became one of the most powerful leaders of history. *Talents used multiply.* The Christian who accepts the challenge to take a new step of faith and become a soul-winner will soon be amazed at his accomplishments.

There is something *you can do* which no one else can ever accomplish — regardless of your age, education, state of health, working hours, or any other circumstance. Can it be said of each of us, "She hath done what she could"?

VIII. PERSONAL REWARDS TO BE ENJOYED.

Those who win souls not only help bring eternal blessings to others but also bring personal rewards to themselves. For instance:

It will promote *happiness and contentment.* Read Psalms 126:5, 6. Everyone wants to be happy. To do so, we must lose ourselves in something greater than ourselves. "Unless above himself he can erect himself, how poor a thing is man!" — Samuel Daniel. Even people of the world feel this and are prompted to do civic and philanthropic works. There is no cause as sublime as Christianity; therefore, promoting it brings the deepest satisfaction. So give yourself away! It will not only help make you happy, but doctors say that it will even improve health.

It is *one way to multiply our lives.* Probably one of the best works ever done by Andrew was bringing Peter to Christ. His faith led to the Lord a worker even greater than himself. An elderly lady said to me: "When I was younger, I didn't fully realize my responsibilities. Now my goal is to teach some talented young woman the truth so that my work will continue long after I am gone." Such a noble ambition. And she has since then achieved it.

Winning souls brings *the joy of usefulness.* In 1912 in Chicago there was a newsboy with a withered leg. One day he read of a little girl who had been severely burned, and he offered the skin from his lame leg to save the girl's life. After the skin was taken, he developed pneumonia. Overhearing the doctor say there was no hope for him, he thoughtfully turned to the doctor and said: "Doc, tell her I'm still glad I did it; now I know that I'm good for something." Everyone has a desire to be useful.

It is such a thrill to hear someone say: "If it had not been for you, I would never have known the truth; and I shall be eternally grateful to you."

The sweetest joys will come one day when we reach heaven and see souls who, but for us, would not be there.

IX. WHY NOT?

In view of these thoughts, why is not every Christian busy winning souls? Numerous reasons and excuses have been offered. Space prohibits a discussion of each. However, when all are analyzed and condensed, there are only two basic reasons why Christians are indifferent toward teaching the lost:

Either they are not convinced they must be soul-winners to go to heaven.

Or, they do not really believe that others must obey the gospel to be saved. There may be a tinge of secret skepticism which causes them to think: "Oh, well, everything is going to turn out all right anyhow." Let's read again the warning in II Thessalonians 1:7-9 concerning the fate of those who "obey not the gospel."

Time flies, the grave awaits, hell threatens, and heaven invites. No wonder God says: "Awake thou that sleepest!"

EXERCISE

1. ". . . now it is high time to .... out of ....:
for now is our salvation .... than when we believed." Was this written to Christians? Is salvation a goal toward which we must strive constantly?

YOU CAN BE BEAUTIFUL 87

2. How did the rich man in hades propose that souls be taught? .... Was such possible? .... Was the rich man given a second chance for salvation? .... Does this emphasize the urgency of teaching the lost now?
3. What kind of fishermen did Christ want Peter, James, and John to be? ....
4. Give the four commands included in Matthew 28:18-20: (1) .... (2) .... (3) .... (4) ....
5. Which Scripture speaks of profit and loss? ....
6. When weaker Christians make mistakes, mature children of God should: (1) ignore them, (2) restore them, or (3) condemn them and talk about them to others. Number .... is correct. Scripture. ....
7. What is the primary work of the church? ....
8. How does God say one may have beautiful feet? ....
9. Christians are to "shine as .... in the world, holding for the .... of ...."
10. "He that goeth forth and weepeth, bearing ...., shall doubtless come again with ...., bringing his .... with him."
11. Statistics show that approximately .... souls depart this life each minute.
12. Which Scripture shows that it is necessary for all to obey the gospel? ....

13. List the two reasons given to explain why more Christians are not soul-winners: ....

....

....

FOR THOUGHT OR DISCUSSION

1. A drowsy, indifferent, lukewarm Christian is so distasteful to the Lord that he says: "I will .... thee out of my ...." (Rev. 3:15, 16).
2. What was the sin of the one talent man? (Matt. 25:18-28) .... Must each account for his talent? Does this parable speak of a "no talent" person?

XIII

Sharing God's Beauty Plan

WHEN Christians are awakened to their responsibilities, they will want to share God's wonderful message with others. The very basis of Christianity is sharing. "Share what you have" (Heb. 13:16, R.S.V.). This must be done through a combination of human efforts and divine power.

Such was fittingly demonstrated by Christ as he used a comparatively insignificant lunch of a boy to feed the multitude (Mark 6:34-44). He required his disciples to measure up their own resources and begin with what they had, however small. Then by divine power the few loaves and fishes were shared by all.

I. "HOW MANY LOAVES HAVE YE? GO AND SEE" (Mark 6:38).

Teeming multitudes today are hungering for the bread of life. What do you have which can be used to feed them?

You have the word of God, the most powerful force in the world. Within it lies the power to save souls, transform lives, and revolutionize the entire world.

You have opportunities on every hand. Truly the fields are white unto harvest. You may stand on your porch and view a lifetime of work. Every person you see is a never-dying soul.

You have the ability to use those opportunities.

II. "EVEN I CAN DO THAT."

At the close of our Bible class one day, a lady of eighty-four said: "Show me our tract supply. I will distribute some through the mail. Even I can do that." Let's consider some indirect methods of soul-winning which can be done by everyone regardless of age, education, or circumstances.

Invite and bring others to the services. If you take someone to the place where the seed of the kingdom is sown into his heart, you can be a partner in winning his soul. Whom can we invite? Neighbors, those who have just moved to town, those with whom we work, co-workers in P. T. A., neighborhood children who are not attending anywhere — just anyone! And remember: nearly everybody is very grateful for an invitation, whether he accepts or not; so don't be hesitant. In this, our telephones can be instruments of the Lord. If you cannot "fill the pulpit," do all you can to fill the pews.

Distribute gospel literature. Numerous examples could be cited of those who learned the truth through reading. A Christian woman said: "I don't feel that I am yet prepared to teach others personally; but in the meantime, I want to give books and tracts to as many people as I can."

Visit new members. Christian friendliness often determines whether a babe in Christ remains faithful to the Lord. This helps to strengthen a soul.

Visit delinquent members. In every city, there are probably as many inactive church members as active ones. Just think what it would mean if all these could be re-enlisted in God's service. While we are busy getting people into the front door of the church, many others are slipping out the back door, figuratively speaking. To restore them to duty is to "save a soul from death;" for when one has left the church, he has left the Lord. Everyone has the ability to say sincerely to a negligent Christian: "We have missed you; we are interested in you and want you to come back to the church and to the Lord." Just a realization that someone cares has helped many to return to active duty.

Use your opportunities *at the worship services.* Strangers who come to the services more than likely feel a keen spiritual need. Whether they are met with a spirit of warmth and love, or one of indifference and iciness, may actually be the turning point in their lives. If we spend all our time talking to "our bunch" after services, those who really need us may go away

YOU CAN BE BEAUTIFUL

unnoticed and unhelped. Make a special effort to meet visitors and to be friendly.

Visit newcomers to your part of town. This promotes goodwill for the church, helps to locate delinquent Christians, and makes contacts with those who are searching for the truth.

III. IS YOUR HOME GOD'S WORKSHOP?

Many mothers who must spend so much time at home have said: "But there is nothing I can do; I'll just have to wait until my children are grown before I can teach others." Consider your home as God's workshop, and think of all the things that can be done there to help sow the seed of the kingdom.

Teaching your own children (and husband, if he is not a Christian) is surely a part of soul-winning and is a vital work, as mentioned elsewhere in our lessons. Though working for the Lord begins at home, it surely does not end there. Your home can serve as a center which radiates light and love to so many others.

Have you ever gathered the neighborhood children into your home for a Bible story? Flannelgraph equipment, blackboards, and other teaching aids can be used at home as well as in the classroom, whether you teach regularly or not.

Have you ever used your morning coffee break to talk to a neighbor about her soul?

Have you ever used your home for someone else to teach a Bible class to your friends and neighbors?

A Christian woman said: "I must be at home so much with my small children; but I have determined to give to each person who knocks at my door — salesmen, delivery boys, or anyone else — a tract and an invitation to worship."

How often has your home been used for some kind of refreshments following the worship services to help encourage new members, weak members, or those who are not yet Christians? Mothers, the spirit of hospitality depends primarily on you. Are social gatherings planned with a specific aim of doing good, or do we spend all our efforts on special friends only?

7. Yes, our homes can be God's workshop, and opportunities are on every hand. Be alert to them, and you will think of many additional things you can do.

IV. TWO "MUSTS" OF DIRECT PERSONAL TEACHING.

Many Christians have said: "I can do some things, but I just cannot personally teach the Bible to another." Perhaps you can do more than you think. If space permitted, we could discuss many "do's" and "don'ts" of soul-winning; however, most of these can be summarized under two "musts." These apply whether teaching one person or several at a time. And remember: one is a big audience.

We must know something to teach. This does not mean that we must know everything. This is what some are waiting on; but if they will begin to use the knowledge they have, their knowledge will increase.

(1) Plan a definite course of study and use a study guide. This will give more confidence and courage than any other one thing. Many people think of personal teaching in terms of going into the midst of people as an open target. Such need not be true. A planned line of thought keeps the study organized. There are numbers of helps now available — cottage Bible class material, correspondence courses, tracts, books, and other aids.

(2) Then familiarize yourself with related Scriptures which may be brought up. Mark your Bible in every helpful way, and keep in your Bible lists of Scriptures on major topics.

(3) Take your concordance or other study helps that you may need for reference.

(4) Understand that you are not expected to know everything and that others are oftentimes put at ease when you say: "I don't know, but let's find the answer to that and discuss it again at a future time." Each new question which arises prompts us to study and to increase our own knowledge.

We must have the right attitude. Many with superior Bible knowledge have failed as soul-winners because of unchristian attitudes. If we keep our attitudes right, then we can grow in knowledge and become powerful workers for the Lord. We must have an attitude of:

(1) Love for souls. If we do, that love will shine through everything we do and say. Some may love an argument and have little love for another's soul. It is possible to win an argument and yet lose the soul. Those who do not truly love the souls of others should never discuss the Bible until their own attitudes are corrected.

(2) Humility. How inconsistent to manifest unchristian arrogance while trying to spread Christianity.

(3) Prayer. Pray before an appointment or visit. Have you learned the value of silent prayer, both before an appointment or during one? Pray with the prospect; it will do something for him or her that nothing else will.

(4) Sympathy. Put yourself in the other person's place and realize that if you had been taught as she was, you would believe and feel just as she does.

(5) A positive attitude. An attitude of kindness and love does not mean a spirit of compromise. Some fail as soul-winners because they do not possess enough faith and firmness to disagree with another and stand staunchly for Bible truths.

PERSONAL EXAMINATION ON SOUL-WINNING

To help us glimpse a vision of our responsibilities and possibilities in the field of soul-winning, consider the following questions:

1. *Do you believe that you have the ability to do the following things:*

    (1) Personally teach a person what to do to be saved? Yes ( ) No ( ) Have you made an effort lately to do so? Yes ( ) No ( )

    (2) Pass out books or tracts that will teach another how to become a Christian? Yes ( ) No ( ) How long has it been since you have done so? ....

YOU CAN BE BEAUTIFUL

(3) Invite your friends to the services? Yes ( ) No ( ) Have you lately invited someone who is not a Christian? Yes ( ) No ( )

(4) Bring others to the services in your car? Yes ( ) No ( ) Have you brought anyone lately? Yes ( ) No ( )

(5) Invite a group into your home for a class taught by someone else? Yes ( ) No ( ) Have you ever made an effort to arrange such a class? Yes ( ) No ( )

(6) Visit members out of duty and express an interest in them? Yes ( ) No ( ) Have you ever made a visit of this kind? Yes ( ) No ( )

(7) Visit new members? Yes ( ) No ( ) Do you ever take the names of new members and call on them without being especially requested to do so? Yes ( ) No ( )

(8) Visit those who have just moved to your section of town and invite them to worship? Yes ( ) No ( ) Have you ever made such a visit? Yes ( ) No ( )

(9) Invite new members into your home to help them get acquainted? Yes ( ) No ( )

(10) Greet strangers at church? Yes ( ) No ( ) Do you think such has any influence at all on whether they may later be led to become Christians? Yes ( ) No ( )

(11) Invite prospects to your home for a brief social following the services? Yes ( ) No ( ) Do you think this would be a means of helping to sow the seed of the kingdom into their hearts? Yes ( ) No ( ) Have you ever done this? Yes ( ) No ( )

2. If the above questions reveal that you are not very active as a soul-winner, *examine yourself and check the reasons:*
( ) Do not think it is your duty.

( ) Do not know enough about the Bible to teach it to others.
( ) A lack of love for souls.
( ) A lack of faith — do not believe deep down in your heart that it is necessary for everyone to obey the gospel to be saved.
( ) Believe that it is a work enjoined only on preachers and elders.
( ) Just too busy to put forth the effort.
( ) Feel that you do not have the ability. If so, re-examine the above list of things and see how many of them you can do.
( ) Afraid to say anything for fear of saying the wrong thing.
( ) Other reasons.

3. How many people do you feel you have had a part in personally teaching to become a Christian? ....

4. Does the Bible teach that it is the responsibility of every Christian to teach the gospel to others? Yes ( ) No ( )

5. At the present time, are you making a special effort to influence some specific person to become a Christian? Yes ( ) No ( )